STOP Feeding Your CANCER

STOP Feeding Your CANCER

One Doctor's Journey

DR JOHN KELLY

PENTHEUM

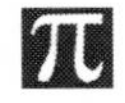

Published 2014 by Pentheum Press,
2 Lower Kennelsfort Road, Palmerstown Village, Dublin 20
Email: pentheumpress@gmail.com

Paperback 978-0-9927798-6-3
Ebook – ePub format 978-0-9927798-7-0
Ebook – mobi format 978-0-9927798-8-7

A CIP catalogue record for this book is
available from the British Library.

Produced by Kazoo Publishing Services
222 Beech Park, Lucan, Co. Dublin
www.kazoopublishing.com

Cover design by Red Rattle Design
Printed by CPI, England

Dedication

To my patients, friends all, who empowered this book.

And to the memory of my brother, with love and respect.

"Two roads diverged in a wood, and I—
I took the one less traveled by,
And that has made all the difference."

ROBERT FROST, "THE ROAD NOT TAKEN"

Contents

Preface

As you will see from page one, this book is autobiographical in that it relates one doctor's experience of the challenge of cancer. In more than 40 years as a general practitioner I have encountered the illness in all its forms and in all its complexity on an almost daily basis, and I have learned much about patients' responses, specialist treatments and situation outcomes. Cancer has visited my own family and, like so many others, I have personally dealt with the stress it brings to lives, and with the frequently helpless confusion. Patients' first reactions on hearing their diagnoses are consistent. Alarm and distress are compounded by ignorance. The headlines about cancer are well known and circulated in the popular press: it is virulent, it is often indiscriminately fatal and treatments are complex and often brutal. Progress towards "the cure" is being made, of course. Progressively our deeper understanding of the scientific basis of life brings forward new variations of treatment, and these are occasionally unveiled at esteemed medical symposia or in the pages of peer-reviewed specialist journals like *The Lancet* or the *British Medical Journal.* But in my experience patients in crisis tend not to read limited-distribution specialist magazines, and if they did I'm not sure they would find solace or indeed clarity in their pages. Currently, there are fortunes being spent on cancer research in hundreds of laboratories and institutions. Importantly, two long, intricate studies of the relationship between nutrition – i.e. food intake – and cancer have reached a kind of conclusion. One, the Harvard School of Public Health report, has indicated a troubling link between the consumption of red meat and dairy products and early death. The other, known as EPIC, the French-English joint venture European Prospective Investigation into Cancer and Nutrition, which gathered data from over half a million volunteers in ten countries over a decade, might best be described as a "lifestyle study". Its results, although not yet fully collated, indicate fundamental contradictions to the Harvard report, prospectively going so far as to upend the long-held conviction that vegetarians live longer, healthier lives than frequent meat-eaters.

The poorly coordinated dissemination of these reports (which often use fundamentally different review techniques) and the contradictions and confusion they give rise to are more than unfortunate, I believe: they are divisive. They cloud the average person's understanding of progress in cancer treatment and recovery and deepen a sense of helplessness in the face of what society has come to see as the unshakeable public enemy No. 1. In the din of contradictory reports and the proliferation of knee-jerk "alternative remedy" responses, some key truths become buried. One such truth is the key to this book. Today's studies – by Harvard and EPIC and the many charity-funded cancer organisations – are unquestionably noble and well-intentioned. But it is regrettable that they are not more clearly aligned with a forensic study published a decade ago that established beyond any reasonable doubt the link between the consumption of animal protein and cancer growth. The work I am referring to is Professor T. Colin Campbell's *The China Study*, which was published in 2005. Campbell is emeritus professor of nutrition at Cornell University and had been exploring the link between meat and cancer cell growth for more than twenty years, initially publishing his findings in peer-reviewed scientific journals that demand the kind of critical-thinking criteria essential to establishing a valid reappraisal of the status quo. Campbell's careful experiments indicated one bald conclusion: that the favourite food of cancer cells happens to be animal protein; ergo, reduction or elimination of animal protein in the human diet stops cancer cell growth. When Campbell published *The China Study*, it was his intention to use the book as a vehicle to bring his findings to the attention of the general public, and especially to those actually suffering from cancer. One would have thought that the detailed research he carried out in preparation for his book would have been sufficient to persuade people to fundamentally readdress their food habits, or at least to have stimulated a more focused and unified international research accord by cancer specialists. The fact that neither happened, that no cultural changes in food marketing or consumption ensued and that no headline unified review efforts were made by the medical science community, was surprising. Indeed, given the implications in terms of health management in an economically stressed and ever-shrinking world, the failure of the medical profession to coordinate a response in a publicized effort to refute or confirm his findings is to my mind something of an embarrassment.

It is because Professor Campbell was not entirely

successful in getting his message across that I began this book. I read and reread his thesis – sceptically, open-heartedly, every which way – and I found myself unable to ignore the importance of the science or the urgency of the message. I was not swayed by any personal prejudice or predisposition: I had no gripe with meat eaters, nor a committed faith in the promised benefits of strict vegetarianism. But facts are facts, and Campbell's records stand up to any scrutiny. Compelled to engage with his findings, I considered my own modest straw-poll study. What, I wondered, would be the fate of my cancer patients if they followed Campbell's study and rigorously adopted the animal-protein-free diet he advocated? Let me stress that as a medical practitioner committed to the well-being of all my patients I was not for a moment contemplating discouraging them from conventional cancer treatments or the wisdom of their specialists. I can claim no special expertise in cancer; but the key remedial findings in *The China Study* and Campbell's potentially corrective indicators appeared so credible – indeed provable – that I felt I could not let the matter rest. The fact that scientists responded so stodgily, that so few who hold influence within the medical community appeared to be interested in Campbell's radical rethinking of cancer treatment, stirred me to immediately take up the challenge.

Let me emphasize here the unbiased, if not outright wary, nature of my own investigation, which will unfold in these pages. When I set up my informal trials with cancer patients selected from my practice, I was aware this would involve neither the number of subject-patients nor the kind of empirical recording standards that represent a full-scale conventional, clinical trial. But I wasn't after that. I was, in the first instance, primarily attempting to gather enough evidence to convince myself where the truth lay. As with any doctor on the frontline of health care, I had seen too much suffering and too many lives cut short by cancer to be blasé about the disease. My reasoning was that any study that proposed widespread remedial value *demanded* the most rigorous and transparent field-testing.

So I proceeded with my own study, with my patients' help. As it turned out I had not long to wait before positive feedback began to come my way. My first pleasant surprise was that most of the patients who participated in the trial reported feeling a good deal better after just weeks of being on an animal-protein-free diet. I was cautious, assuming first the probability of a psychosomatic effect resulting from the pep talk I had given each patient prior to entering the trial. Nevertheless the overwhelming positivity gave both the patients and me a certain amount of encouragement.

Compliance, however, proved to be the major stumbling block with the trial. This I had anticipated. The human factor in informal trials must always be taken into account, and I understood that giving up favourite foods was going to be difficult for patients. It was apparent to me that all but the most highly motivated found sticking the course tough. These patients were of course also in the care of oncologists – conventionally trained cancer consultants. The fact that there was no support forthcoming from their cancer specialists added greatly to the problems of the trial, with the result that a great many participants faltered in spite of all my efforts and either reverted to their previous eating habits or adhered to the diet only sporadically. This at first seemed a considerable setback. But I realized that it also meant that those who remained in the trial were excellent subjects due to their exceptional motivation and commitment to strictly following the diet. What I lost in quantity, therefore, I made up for in quality.

Most of the patients who remained in the trial were suffering from advanced cancer and had poor long-term prognoses. What they had in common was that, although they were all suffering from serious forms of cancer, their vital organs were intact and functional. And so we soldiered on.

What transpired was startling. Sometimes simplification seems alien to science, and medicine in particular. We come to expect complexity in the modern world and we overlook the simple principle of cause and effect. Simply put, once these patients adhered to the diet, their cancers stopped growing and they could get back to their normal lives.

My trial spanned eight years, since my first encounter with Professor Campbell's work. After those eight years, I have one very striking statistic. I can claim that with the exception of cancer of the pancreas, of which much later, not one of the cancer patients who have been on an animal-protein-free diet and remained faithful to it have died from their disease. This presents us with a truly *vital* statistic, because all it takes is a single failure, one lost patient, for my experimental house of cards to come tumbling down.

"Preposterous!" is what cancer specialists generally said when they heard about my trial. "That just couldn't be true." My riposte was that they should do their own research and make their judgement then. I found these encounters with specialists disturbing, not because my feelings were hurt, but because they gave me an indication of the likely reaction I would get from the medical profession when the results of my rather suburban trial were finally published. It was when attempting to put together a plan of action on how best to overcome the complacency of cancer specialists towards Colin Campbell's ideas that thoughts of outsiders like Lyall Watson came into my head. On my bookshelves I saw two of his books, *Supernature* and *Lifetide*. Watson was an anthropologist and biologist who had influenced an entire generation with subject matter that was very much on the grey edge of science. He wrote on taboo subjects such as intuition, telepathy and shamanic magic, and he made those arcane subjects accessible to a wide audience that earlier respected writers – authors like the scholar Robert Graves or the psychologist Abraham Maslow – had failed to win. He struck a note that resonated with people, allowing them to discover things about themselves and their environment that were previously overlooked. Although scientists regarded his work as speculative, they at least paid attention. He made mistakes (he was provably wrong in one famous anthropological guess) but when he died, the *New York Times* obituary saluted him as a maverick, scientific polymath – a significant summary when one understands that "polymath" comes from the Greek polymathēs, meaning "having learned much". If Lyall Watson were alive today I am sure he would not think my work deluded.

I have only one taboo subject to talk about here, and the book in your hands shares the same objective Watson had, which is to tackle the limitations of convention, stimulate debate and speed up the search for the truth. No author who embarks on a book can foresee its final destination. For the author each work is a voyage of discovery fated to end in success or failure, in which he can only pledge to do his best. Herein I offer you the best of my labours over the last decade. The destination I hope for is an increased, shared awareness of the powers we all have – not hidden or esoteric in any way, but rather readily, easily accessible – to face and overcome challenges, and to help ourselves to heal.

Dr John Kelly, MB
Dublin, Summer 2014

1

Important News About Cancer

"All truths are easy to understand once they are discovered.The point is to discover them."

— GALILEO

THE STORY OF THE TWO PADDIES

What may come to be viewed as a major advance in the treatment of cancer was presented to me over lunch on the day my good friend Paddy was buried. I had known Paddy for a very long time and as I sat alone in the hotel restaurant I was thinking that the world would be a lonelier place without him. Although he had been 70 years old when he died of cancer, I was not ready for him to go, as I had always expected that he would live to a ripe old age. His father had died at the age of 105 and his mother had lived until she was almost 90. It seemed to me that Paddy's genes had somehow let him down.

Our friendship went back to our college days. We had attended the same university, where he studied accountancy and I medicine. Ours was an unlikely friendship, as on the surface we appeared to differ from each other considerably.

The initial impression one might have had of Paddy was that he was a well-mannered, conservative person, someone whom one could count upon to behave properly at all times. He had a wide circle of friends that fit well with his public persona, most of whom seemed to know a very different side of Paddy than the one I knew. To me he was a man who was uniquely capable of defying the very establishment he appeared to epitomize. He wasn't quite a gangster, but he enjoyed thumbing his nose at authority.

During our college years our relationship centred mostly on going horse racing together, and we attended practically all of the Saturday race meetings that took place in the Dublin area. He had grown up in a small town in rural Ireland and knew a lot about horses. Among his acquaintances were trainers, jockeys and owners whom he made a point of bumping into at race meetings, to gather some tips. The result was that we sometimes managed to have quite a few winners. As gamblers go, I wasn't in the same league as Paddy. He was the astute, professional betting man, always reading the signs and prepared to wait for the right race and the right moment before placing his bet. I was the sort of punter on whom the bookmakers thrived, as I had a tendency to place a bet on every race just for the hell of it. As a result I had the annoying habit of running out of money long before Paddy did, sometimes very early on in the college term.

Occasionally even Paddy's luck would run out, and when such disaster struck we would cut down on expenses by hitching lifts to the racetrack and, whenever the opportunity presented itself, even clambering over the perimeter walls to avoid paying the entrance fee. This trickery became something of an enjoyable pastime. The conservative, immaculately dressed Paddy always took the lead in these activities, while

I was happy to follow. Paddy had impeccable timing and we were invariably successful. It was simply a matter of looking over the wall and noting the position of the white-coated officials inside the course; then over we would go. Even if the officials spotted us, we always managed to evade capture, as by the time they arrived at the scene of the crime we had blended into the crowd. A misplaced sense of propriety meant the white-coated men were loath to confront the toffish, elegant racing enthusiasts watching the horses at the parade ring.

Sitting in the hotel after the funeral, waiting for the reception to begin, I smiled to myself as all these memories came flooding back. It wasn't just racing. I remembered a crisp, sunny Saturday morning many years ago. Paddy had telephoned to ask if I was interested in going to the rugby international between Ireland and England that was taking place in Dublin that day. The match was sold-out and, naturally, given our social standing, we had no tickets. As security is normally very tight at such games I didn't hold much hope for our chances of gaining entry, but as I had no plans I said I would go along. Paddy was in top form that morning and relished the challenge. No discussion took place about how we might gain entrance and the only preparation Paddy made was to cut out two pieces of card so that they vaguely resembled tickets. An hour or so before the match was due to start we stood near the turnstiles and watched the people streaming into the grounds. There was a ticket collector at each turnstile, inside a little kiosk, and the people queued up to pass their tickets through a small hatch. We noticed that the collector at kiosk number two was taking the tickets and placing them somewhat carelessly in a little pile just inside the hatch, allowing the punters to pass through into the stadium more quickly than the fellows manning the other kiosks.

Just as I was thinking we had no hope, Paddy leaned over and whispered into my ear, "This should be easy." He told me to take up a position near the front of the queue of the adjoining turnstile and he approached kiosk number two. The trick in all his escapades was to distract his victim. His strategy was not to look at the person directly in the eyes but at a spot in the middle of their forehead. When done properly this has a slightly distracting effect and it was as he did this that Paddy passed the piece of cardboard into the collector's hand and grabbed a bunch of tickets from the pile just inside that hatch. Then he stepped backwards and to the side while the ticket collector struggled to get out of his kiosk. Paddy slipped ahead of me at the front of the adjoining queue, passing the bunch of stolen tickets – save one – into my hand. He used the remaining one to pass through turnstile number three into the stadium. It was all over in a matter of seconds.

In the melee that followed, with Paddy safely inside the grounds, I quietly withdrew out of harm's way and proceeded to an area just outside the stadium gates where touts and people trying to sell surplus tickets usually gathered. I sold a number of the tickets to a couple of rich-looking folk and distributed the rest of them Robin Hood-style to those I thought looked most deserving. I gave two to a very pretty girl who was standing with her boyfriend. In those days the grateful smile of a pretty girl was payment enough for anything.

ANOTHER PADDY

What has all this got to do with cancer, you might ask.

Well, it was at the reception after Paddy's funeral that I met another friend called Paddy. People were beginning to take their places at tables, when I felt a tap on my shoulder and this other Paddy sat down beside me. He too had been a fellow student during my college years and he had been a very good friend of the deceased Paddy. I hadn't seen him for a very long time. This Paddy had the reputation of being one of the brightest students in college and had gone on to become a very distinguished professor of genetics. At the time of the funeral he was already something of an icon in Irish science. As our paths had rarely crossed over the years, I was delighted to meet him again.

While this second Paddy and I got on fairly well, we had never been very close friends; there had always been a little tension between us. Paddy had been one of the deceased Paddy's more respectable friends and he had a way of looking at me that suggested he did not entirely trust me. It wasn't that we didn't like each other, but there was a sort of competitive mistrust between us that became particularly evident when we famously undertook a car journey together across the United States. The trip had been organized to be more or less non-stop, but we had squabbled so much about which route to take that we were in real danger of going around in circles. Our adventure could have ended badly, but instead it evolved into something of a good-natured game, thanks largely to the constant good humour and diplomatic skills of Roderick, the third companion-driver on that journey.

The idea of the trip had come about in a Dublin pub some months previously. I had been explaining that I was committed to go to my sister's wedding in Los Angeles when Paddy mentioned that it had always been one of his ambitions to drive across the States from New York to LA. He suggested that we all go to the wedding. Having studied at Cornell University he had useful stateside contacts and explained how there were always people wanting their cars transported from east to west coast and that he could probably arrange something. And that's how our improbable trip came about: whimsically arranged in a pub on a wet Saturday afternoon in 1962, with no consideration of anything beyond Destination LA.

Now, all these years later, here was Paddy sitting beside me, and it was plain from his body language and the smiles on both our faces that any differences between us had been long since forgotten. We had lost an old friend and we found solace in our reminiscences: true friends are rare; old friends are gold.

The fact that Paddy was now a famous geneticist prompted me to tease him a little, and I complained about treacherous genes. It was unacceptable, I said, that our dear friend died at such a relatively young age when there was a history of longevity in his family. Paddy, never one to suffer fools, just shrugged his shoulders. "If you want to know more about cancer, you should read *The China Study*," he said. I had never heard of *The China Study*. He explained how a friend of his, Colin Campbell, who had been professor of nutrition at Cornell when Paddy was there doing postgraduate work, had written a book about cancer. Paddy had found the book interesting and he looked me straight in the eye and said he would value my opinion on it. He wrote the details on the back of one of his business cards and smiled at me in a way that reminded me of how he used to smile when he was trying to get the better of me in an argument. That was the end of the conversation. Other people joined us at the table and we did not speak on the subject again.

Hours after I left the reception, I was still thinking about our conversation. I was flattered and intrigued that Paddy should have asked me to read and evaluate Professor Campbell's book, but I also felt wary. Paddy knew my life story well enough, and by his standards (I assumed) I would have been something of an underachiever as far as medicine was concerned. Instead of specializing after medical school I had spent seven years wandering around the world working in different countries. This had been my ambition since childhood. I had graduated in Ireland and then worked in the United States and France before giving in to my wanderlust. I had gone to sea, circumnavigating the world as a ship's doctor on a cadet-training vessel. After that, following a short spell working in a psychiatric hospital in Ireland, I met a Mauritian girl and decided to settle in Mauritius. I got married there, but because I had no specialist training to speak of and as there was an oversupply of doctors in Mauritius at the time, I had little option but to return to Ireland and set up in primary care medicine as a general practitioner. Serendipity plays strange games with our lives, and Ireland turned out to be a place of fulfilment for me. I raised a family, made good friends and was happy to remain here and, in that time-honoured cliché, settle down. Paddy would have known about my regular practice but he also knew my wandering ways and stubborn nature and, I reasoned, would hardly have been impressed.

It puzzled me, therefore, that he was soliciting an opinion from me on *The China Study*. Without question he had many esteemed colleagues who were much more knowledgeable about cancer than I. Their specialized opinions surely carried weight. They were the professors with tenure, the research-funded scientists, the scions of the great American health institutions.

The day after the funeral I went to the local bookshop to purchase a copy of *The China Study*. He had spoken of it as though it was a seminal work, and I assumed that I would easily pick up a copy. But, to my great surprise, no one at the bookstore had ever heard of it. Paddy must have anticipated the obstacles I might encounter, because a few days later I received a large envelope in the post with copious information about Professor Campbell and the nutritional studies that formed the basis of his book. Paddy's accompanying note said, "See what you make of it. It's outside my field of expertise, but perhaps you can take it to the next level." He was obviously keen that I should read the book, and when I pushed aside the flattery, I began to suspect that *The China Study* was niggling at his conscience, that he had found something in its contents that irked or troubled him as a geneticist and that he was intent on passing the problem on to someone else.

When I finally got the book and read it, I was impressed. Campbell's account, though scientifically detailed, was linear, coherent and credible, and I found I could identify with many casebooks, issues and conclusions based on my own experience and on my everyday encounters in the surgery. I realized also that Paddy, being familiar with my instinctively inquisitive nature, would probably have anticipated my response to the book. But the pointedness of his appeal for my opinion still seemed strange to me. In the upper echelons of the medical world, the opinion of a general practitioner doesn't count for much. The implications of Campbell's work in terms of demanding a radical review of cancer treatment were so great that I could imagine an ambitious geneticist like Paddy rattling every door, querying commentaries, urging revolutionary action at the National Institutes of Health. After all, there were precedents. When the true breakthrough in antibiotics occurred in the twentieth century, no holds were barred in conquering such terrible diseases as TB. Salk's work on polio received enormous support and encouragement. The scourge of smallpox had been eradicated entirely because a wide community of practitioners got behind committed medical visionaries. Surely Colin Campbell's groundbreaking statistics were comparable to the great revelations of streptomycin as an effective cure for TB or Salk's IPV polio vaccine? Surely Paddy had little trouble exciting others who ranked highly in the medical community to engage with Campbell's initiative?

Later that week I got my answer when I met up with a professor of medicine whom I knew from one of Dublin's medical schools. I was hitting a bucket of golf balls at the driving range and he was practising in the booth next to mine. We chatted and I casually brought up *The China Study*. He listened briefly and then stopped me in mid-sentence to declare dismissively that he had never heard of it. Rather impatiently he informed me that although Colin Campbell might be a professor of nutrition at a very prestigious university, he was no medical specialist. Furthermore, he opined, as a professor of nutrition such people as Campbell were among the most dangerous, as they did not have expertise necessary to make judgements on medical matters. Lay people were vulnerable, he said, because they could be tempted to believe the kind of unqualified claims people like Campbell made. In his opinion, if there was any truth in what Campbell wrote, "it's up to the appropriate medical specialists to follow it up."

That was it, subject closed. My professor friend went on hitting his golf balls as if nothing of consequence had passed between us. He had no more words of wisdom, but what he had said helped me to understand why Paddy had asked me to read *The China Study*. It was precisely because I was not a specialist that he focused on me. *I* was not constrained by the politics or conservatism of the higher medical establishment. I was neither cynical nor gullible, nor was I trying to protect a tenure or toe any party lines. I was independent-minded and I was in daily contact with ordinary patients struggling with extraordinary ailments. I was involved, but my inquisitiveness matched my discipline. And this meant I might have an open mind.

WHAT PROFESSOR CAMPBELL HAD TO SAY

After reading the first few pages of *The China Study* it was clear that Colin Campbell was neither a charlatan nor a deluded fanatic. He was a scientist with a fascinating story to tell. His work on cancer began in the 1960s when he had worked on an aid programme in the Philippines. At that time, along with serious malnutrition, an unusually high rate of liver cancer existed among children in the country. The cause of the liver cancer was attributed to the fact that a fungus which produced a highly carcinogenic substance had contaminated the peanut crop. A very strange statistic came to the attention of the researchers. They discovered that although children from all sections of the community ate peanuts, it was predominantly the children from wealthy families who died of liver cancer. When they attempted to explain this, they found that apart from financial circumstances, the principal discernible difference between the two groups of children was that those coming from wealthy families ate a lot of animal protein. In stark contrast, the children from poorer families consumed practically none. This finding sparked the interest of Professor Campbell.

His curiosity was further aroused when he read an article published in a little-known medical journal from India. This article also suggested that animal protein might be associated with liver cancer. The Indian researchers had attempted to determine what effect, if any, animal protein might have on liver cancer in rats. The rats used in the experiment became prone to cancer when given aflatoxin, the very same carcinogen that had contaminated peanut production in the Philippines. In parallel, two groups of these rats were given diets containing either 20 per cent or 5 per cent animal protein. Over a period of 100 weeks it was determined that all of the rats that had received the diet high in animal protein had died or were dying of cancer. But, notably, not a single rat in the group on a low-animal-protein diet developed the disease. The contrast between the two study cases was quite astonishing. In isolation, each story presented a curious, random finding; viewed together, they presented indications of a significant pattern.

Going on the evidence of the published material, it seems few people read the report from India; and, among those engaged in prominent health-related research institutions, it appears only Professor Campbell paid much attention. Inspired by the Indian lab study and by what he himself had experienced in the Philippines, Campbell decided to set up his own research plan. He used similar cancer-prone rats and experimented with diets containing the same 20 per cent dairy protein (casein) and 5 per cent dairy protein. After 100 weeks, all of the rats in the 20 per cent group were either dead or dying of cancer, while none of those in the 5 per cent group were. He experimented further with some of the rats that had already developed cancer, replacing their 20 per cent dairy-protein diet with one that had less than 5 per cent, and found that the cancers immediately stopped growing and began to recede. His own research findings provided him with first-hand evidence that animal protein played a key role in the growth of cancer.

Knowing that he was on to something important, Campbell continued his research into other types of protein, with further significant results. He discovered that not all proteins were the same. In his lab studies it became clear that vegetable proteins did not promote cancer, even when eaten in very large amounts. Another major finding was that if the animal-protein intake was below 5 per cent the promotion of cancer did not appear to occur. It began to seem evident that animal protein was an essential food of cancer cells and that it allowed them to replicate. Another study concluded that once the healthy cells had utilized the animal protein, the leftovers were then consumed by the cancer cells. Therefore, keeping the amount of animal protein in the diet below 5 per cent was all that was necessary to stop cancers from growing. No leftovers meant no food for the cancer cells.

The facts began to accumulate for Campbell, leaving inescapable deductions. Animal-protein consumption was problematic beyond doubt. While a diet of up to 5 per cent animal protein may well be safe, he inferred, it might perhaps be wiser for people suffering from aggressive cancers to reduce their animal-protein intake to considerably less than 5 per cent, indeed to consider eliminating it altogether. From comprehensive published studies over many decades worldwide, there was one undisputed fact: humans can manage very well without any animal protein in their diet. One can remain in good health by eating only the proteins contained in fish, whole grains, pulses, beans, vegetables, fruit and nuts. Humankind evolved as a species eating these foods. As modern man has become increasingly wealthy, he has organized and developed his skills in animal husbandry, exploitation and marketing. Consequently he has broadened his diet and eaten more meat. As he has done so, the prevalence of cancer has increased. One might speculate that cancer is a cruel symptom of affluence.

All of these remarkable conclusions were coming together in Professor Campbell's mind. With the presumption, scientifically well founded, that what pertained in rats was also likely to be relevant to humans, all that now remained was to embark on further research, using human subjects, to prove that this was indeed the case.

2

The Myth of Infallibility

"Every great advance in natural knowledge has involved the absolute rejection of authority."

– THOMAS HUXLEY

NOT INTERESTED

My first move after reading *The China Study* was to explore what my colleagues in general practice would have to say about it. I shared with them my enthusiasm about Campbell's rigorous experiments with rats and the story of how my esteemed geneticist friend had found his book plausible. My colleagues were profoundly unimpressed, the unanimous opinion being that with so much research on cancer already taking place under the auspices of such great institutions as America's National Institutes of Health (NIH), it was most improbable that a vital association between animal protein and cancer could have gone unnoticed. This dismissive reaction did not come as much of a surprise. I knew that most doctors had become increasingly sceptical of such claims, as books espousing various diets purporting to help cure cancer had become commonplace, and claims that vitamins and various supplements might also be useful constantly featured in the media. In most instances, however, such claims were backed up with little more than skimpy anecdotal evidence, and when put to the test they were found to be of little benefit. I was a sceptic myself and I realized that, had it not been for Paddy the geneticist, I would never have considered the thesis contained in *The China Study*.

I was therefore neither offended nor deterred by the reaction of my colleagues. On the other hand, I was a little sad. The status quo being what it is, it was clear they regarded their qualitative evaluations as irrelevant. The view of Professor Campbell or Paddy the geneticist might have mattered, but since neither of them were cancer specialists, their take on the matter was valueless. My colleagues' sentiments deferred entirely to the so-called experts in the field; there could be no argument with that.

In the weeks that followed those exchanges I had, by chance, the opportunity to talk about the book with a well-established cancer specialist. His response was somewhat depressing. He had, he said, never heard of Professor Campbell or *The China Study*. Indeed, his tone of voice quickly told me he wasn't interested. He briefly argued that since he hadn't heard of the book, it was most unlikely to contain anything of value. He huffed a little and baldly expressed surprise that I should allow myself to be taken in by it. When I told him that I already had a couple of patients starting the diet as part of an informal test, he warned me of the possible medico-legal issues that could arise should anything go wrong. I was defensive, I suppose, and offered him my copy of *The China Study* so that he could judge the research for himself. He declined. He was too busy, he said, and even if he were interested, funding for a structured follow-up project – even one endorsed by as important a specialist as himself – would almost certainly not be forthcoming. The world of institutional medicine, it seemed, had its time-tested ways and was not to be challenged.

It was all quite discouraging and I felt pushed to quit. I think I would have at that point had it not been for the fact that it was Paddy the geneticist, my old sparring partner, who had set the challenge. It was boyish and stubborn, I know, but there was an underlying mutual respect between us that made his introduction of the issue electrifying. My encounter with the cancer specialist therefore had the effect of making me redouble my efforts. My mind went into overdrive and I made the decision to stick to my task. Specialists, after all, could be wrong. I thought of Barry Marshall and Robin Warren, the microbiologists in Australia who had been ridiculed when they suggested that the bacterium *Helicobacter pylori* might play a role in the development of peptic ulcers. In spite of resistance from their colleagues, they had persevered, and after eight years they were awarded the Nobel Prize.

In fact doctors have quite a history of being wrong and of staying wrong for a very long time. The practice of bloodletting is a case in point. This practice originated in the ancient civilizations of Egypt and Greece and it is an illustration, not alone of how wrong doctors can be, but also of how long they can remain in error. Bloodletting is believed to have originated when doctors observed how women felt considerably better after menstruation. In ancient times there was little understanding of human anatomy or physiology. It was not unreasonable to suppose that if menstruation could make women feel better, then perhaps bleeding might also be useful when people felt unwell as a result of disease. The practice was implemented and deemed appropriate and it continued for thousands of years as an accepted treatment for many and diverse diseases. These included heart failure, pneumonia, anaemia, fever, headaches, depression – indeed all forms of neuroses – and even extended to assisting the healing of broken bones. As the procedure involved a considerable amount of skill, bloodletting became an important medical specialty. These "specialists" were usually summoned to the bedside of the incapacitated patients by less expert doctors and the cachet of their so-called specialization lent them quite a reputation. A visit by a bloodletting specialist was a sure sign that everything possible was being done for that patient, and somehow this convention successfully masked for centuries the fact that in almost all instances no improvement occurred in the condition of the patients. The truth was that the practice of bloodletting frequently contributed to the cause of death.

Bloodletting as a standard "specialist" medical procedure only came under critical review in the nineteenth century when Louis Pasteur and Robert Koch, two heavyweight scientists nobody could ignore, discovered that microorganisms were responsible for many of the diseases that were being treated by bloodletting. After this revelation, the practice decreased dramatically, and by the early part of the twentieth century it had been almost entirely discredited and abandoned.

The moral of the story is that doctors can sometimes be blind to the errors of their ways. Bloodletting had entered into the belief system of the medical profession in such a way that it became unchallengeable. This was in spite of the fact that any experienced medical professional should have been immediately aware that loss of blood weakened patients and increased the risk of mortality. The "specialist" view was the wrong view.

Today, specialist medicine is at the height of its power and influence because it declares itself to be exclusively science-based, and science, in the popular interpretation, never lies. So the image that contemporary specialist medicine projects – I'm loath to say trades on – is one of near infallibility. This, of course, is partially a social issue. The public wants, is indeed entitled to, the best that medicine has to offer. They want specialists to know everything there is to know about their particular diseases and they want to trust them unequivocally. Such a situation is fraught. With patients continually demanding progress in knowledge and cures, one sees specialists divided between hyper-caution and omnipotence. This is a bind that hampers medicine because it is evident that we are a long way from knowing all there is to know about diseases and a long way from curing many of them, and the inertia imposed upon or conceded to by specialists and experts renders infallibility a dangerous, stubborn myth.

I have little doubt that my friend Paddy knew all of this when he waved the red rag of Campbell's study in front of me. Obviously he had been impressed enough by the research to want to do something about it, but as a fully paid-up member of the exclusive "club of convention", he knew the obstacles he would have encountered had he attempted to promote the book or advance Campbell's theories himself.

My son is astute. He mentioned to me that I should feel flattered that my accomplished friend had chosen to pass an important baton to me. But I told him that our history of competitiveness and the fact that he nearly always came off best made me wonder about other motives. Was Paddy handing me an impossible task, something so outrageous as to be beyond even a pyrrhic victory? But then, I wasn't always outfoxed. I recalled one time I got the better of him. He liked to always be in control, but on our journey across the States we had to pull in for a pit stop to get a broken exhaust pipe repaired. Paddy had fallen asleep on the back seat, so I had the blissful joy of seeing him trapped in the car, elevated on the garage hoist for more than an hour while the pipe was repaired. He had not enjoyed that experience, but I am certain it did him good. I suggested to my son that passing *The China Study* challenge to me was perhaps his way of exacting revenge. My way of trumping him would be to succeed in the task he had set me.

3

The Truth Unfolds

"All truth passes through three stages. First, it is ridiculed. Second, it is violently opposed. Third, it is accepted as self-evident."

– SCHOPENHAUER

IMPARTING TRUTH

The failure of *The China Study* to translate research momentum into efficient, globally coordinated empirical testing was to my mind a tragedy. Though "endorsement" agencies like the *New York Times* reviewed the book favourably, it didn't have an impact on the critical peer-reviewed medical publications, and my own research revealed that few practising doctors had read the book. Clearly its problem was one of badly informed preconceptions, and it had become categorized with the anecdotal tracts that alternative medicine continually offered. In the early 2000s the concept of diet playing an important role in cancer remained very much in the realm of alternative medicine, which in turn sat uncomfortably under the umbrella of dubious New Age thinking. The fact that New Age, despite its crank connotations, embraces such urgent re-evaluations as the neural function discoveries prompted by the likes of Aldous Huxley, Terrence McKenna and John E. Mack is by the by; clearly only medical establishment endorsement had the power to move on Campbell's work. But the obstacles were huge, and moved beyond medical complacency. Think of it. If Campbell's theories proved true, the implications for the global economy were immense. The food and pharmaceutical industries, for starters, would be changed in fundamental and revolutionary ways. Societies would be educated to reorder their values in ways unseen since the benefits of hygiene became the global war cry. I was aware of where Campbell had fallen, and I knew where I might fall. It was an issue of radical universality, an issue of essences, and an issue shrouded in paradox. We trust our doctors. We are now asking them to mistrust themselves.

Imagine doctors universally proclaiming that animal protein makes cancers grow. It would be heresy! Everyone accepts that animal protein is the single most important component in our diet and that its key values – the iron, the A and B vitamins – are essential for the healthy growth and maintenance of all the cells in the body. This "fact" is one of the articles of faith within medicine that nobody in their right mind should dare to challenge. It is outrageous to suggest that in certain circumstances animal product can be seriously bad for us! But the crux of the problem is emotional rather than scientific. Nutritionists have for so long believed that animal protein is beneficial that the very idea that it can do harm seems ludicrous. Redefining animal protein as the favourite food of cancer, and proving that without it a cancer would not thrive or grow, was going to take some work, I knew. My informal general-practice evaluation might not be enough. Transposing those results into a book might risk accusations of yet more anecdotal reportage. But "doing a Hercule

Poirot" in assembling the chain from the Philippines and Indian studies that inspired Campbell at Cornell, through the realities of random patients' lives and treatments, just might nudge the institutional community towards a willingness to change. Life is all about change. I reminded myself as I recorded every patient file and wrote every page of this book that Ireland's first high king, Brian Boru, could never have conceived of a world where television, not tribal war, was the great unifier. And no New World, with all its riches, would ever have been found without Columbus' and Cook's maps. My job was to build a map that might convince the medical profession to look without prejudice at a crippling problem in a new way.

The first person I had to convince of the validity of my case study was myself. I am by nature cautious, as befits all medical practitioners. My first and major concern is for the well-being of my patients, many of whom I regard as friends. I tend not to confront any individual presenting with symptoms in a narrow way, by which I mean that I listen and observe (of course) intently, but also assess in a holistic way, taking a psychosocial overview that embraces the patient's thought processes and lifestyle. This is a diagnostic advantage as it allows not just evaluation of the degree of the disease, but some sense of the potential root or of the factors that have exacerbated a problem. Specialized medicine, not unreasonably, looks to the frontiers of science, concentrating on the molecular and atomic composition of the patient. This approach is of course valid and recognizes the complexity of the human organism. But that complexity enshrines emotional and spiritual issues beyond the remit of the science lab. This has always been central in my thinking: that the fullest organic study must bridge the experience of general practice and the science of the lab. Context is everything, and the distance I observed between the average patient's reality and the clinical function of specialized medicine too often complicated treatment and hampered understanding and resolution.

I know these statements are radical. But in my view it is vital for professional pacemakers to be always reassessing context. History is studded with institutional assumptions that led to wrong tracks and blind alleys. It is astonishing to see how taking a narrow view can stymie the truth. Today, for example, the origins of Egyptian civilization, a bedrock of modern Western civilization, is in critical debate. The accepted academic wisdom for almost two centuries was that the civilization is about 5,000 years old and that the Great Sphinx was built by the Pharaoh Chefren in about 2500 B.C., at a time when the Nile region, once green and naturally fertile, was a desert. The indigenous limestone from which the Sphinx and its companion pyramids were built was, academics said, subject to wind-erosion, hence the distinctive patterns of decay on all the Cairo monuments. It was only in the 1970s that the maverick Egyptologist René Schwaller de Lubicz's evidence for water erosion (which forms a completely different decay "fingerprint" on soft limestone) as the probable cause of the Sphinx's weathering was accepted. Academics were forced to contemplate a civilization far, far older than had been commonly agreed, dating to a time of diluvial tides and a green and fertile Nile Valley.

So much for institutional archaeology. Astronomy and astrophysics, very much the flavour-of-the-month sciences, stand on similarly wobbly foundations. The great modern popularizer of astro studies was the late Sir Patrick Moore, the man who holds the record for the longest continual span broadcasting the same television show, *The Sky at Night*. Moore's meticulous lunar maps were used by NASA in planning the moon landings, and he was knighted for his services to science. But Moore's career, he frequently said, was built on the first science book he'd read, G. F. Chambers' *The Story of the Solar System*, published in 1895. Reading Chambers' book today one is flabbergasted by the assumptions and short cuts. The minor planets of the Kuiper belt beyond Neptune had yet to be discovered, of course, but Chambers excuses all omissions as the mystery of God's ways. His summary of the origins and purpose of the universe handed the issue over to metaphysics, effectively passing the buck. It would take more mavericks like Max Planck, the originator of quantum science theory, (and indeed Moore himself) to open the way for our true understanding of astronomy and the borders of dark matter, dark energy and dark flow that today's visionaries like Stephen Hawking tell us will explain how matter – and we – came into being.

I read as widely and critically as I could before immersing myself in my post-*China Study* experiment. When I felt I'd adequately rationalized the validity of the maverick approach, I considered the framework of my general-practice poll and decided that informality was essential. I must introduce my cancer patients to the concepts put forward by Professor Campbell, urge adherence to an animal-protein-free diet, make no promises and record everything. This exercise proved rewarding, and very early on I saw positive results. Elation was mitigated by the need to consider a sober structure for a book. The goal was clear: I needed to amass case studies and chart results. But I also, more importantly, needed to advertise my patients' experience and lend them a voice. The most important information would be their results and conclusions, not mine. My job was to chart it all, then retreat. But the book, the log of the journey, as it were, was vital. I was no writer, I knew, but the dynamics of a readable, durable book had to be tackled. Would I study genome experiments and the NIH cancer trials and attempt to dissect and challenge them page-by-page, using experience from my surgery? I thought not. My job was to be autobiographical in the simplest sense: to describe my own journey in a common medical situation with everyday patients in layman's terms. The world had had enough of portentous statistics peddlers and snake-oil merchants. Professor Campbell's easy-to-understand, well-tested science deserved an equally clear follow-up.

We kicked off with fingers crossed, but progress was immediate. It was humbling to see the patients' response to the dietary changes I introduced them to. They were getting better, yet they could hardly believe the effect an animal-protein-free life was having. I took my time processing my own response. It was hard to take in, but it seemed that what worked on Campbell's laboratory rats worked on humans. The cases in my surgery multiplied. There was a sense of optimism, then a surge of exaltation. We now had demonstrable evidence that animal protein was required in order for a cancer to grow. I had a conundrum. Initially most of my study patients were happy to credit their progress to some of the treatments their specialists were giving them. This posed a real problem because of their reflex response – sadly, patients became careless with their diet as soon as the cancer showed signs of abating. Clear patterns emerged. Rigorous adherence to the diet showed extraordinary results; those who lapsed suffered relapses and declined in health.

I knew I must persevere and I was fortunate to have the trust of many heroic patients. I knew that, socially, I had failed to engage the interest of fellow doctors, but I now had more than Professor Campbell's study to arrest their attention. I told my patients about this book. The results of the ongoing trials were leading us into new territory, I felt. If word of mouth popularized the book and its findings, the institutional community that had shied away from the challenge in Campbell's book might be stirred to better action.

And so as one, we – my patients and I – soldiered ahead with this work in your hands. Let me stress that I was aware that my research was nowhere near sufficient in itself to convince the mandarins who mould policy at such distinguished agencies as the World Health Organization. The fact is that random cases do not provide the sort of empirical proof that science demands. But my study, informal as it was, became cogent when viewed alongside Professor Campbell's research and, to me, justified further urgent, *targeted* clinical investigation at the very least. It's a challenging fact that established scientific research protocol involves peer review of everything that is published. In practice, this means that new ideas arise only from within the system. My problem, of course, is that I am not, by the accepted definition, a peer. I told my patients: the medical community didn't read Professor Campbell's book, so why should they read mine? They too can only hope that the tide of public opinion that this book might generate can revolutionize entrenched positions.

Regrettably, Colin Campbell found doors closed to him that ought to have been open. He speculated that commercial interests were to blame for the study being ignored by the medical community, and this is indeed deeply troubling. As you meet my patients in the following chapters and consider the medical implications, reflect upon the consequences of a publicly embraced animal-protein-free diet. There is little doubt that the structure of the food industry would change. The chemical companies that produce pharmaceutical cancer treatments would also be challenged. There are billions of dollars tied up in these companies and that means there are many investors who want to protect their investment. Thought must be given to these issues. But such consideration should not take priority over health care. As a medical doctor, I learned the parameters of my civic role early on, and in the workplace my exposure to suffering nurtured in me the kind of empathy we all owe our fellow man. Regardless of the political fallout, it is evident to me that health comes first. My patients are the pioneers of change here and I'd like you to meet them.

4

What Happens in Rats Happens in Humans

"The good god is in the detail."

— GUSTAVE FLAUBERT

CASE STUDIES

Ronan

Ronan was in his mid-sixties when he developed cancer of the colon. He had a passion for sailing and it was during a sailing trip off the coast of England that he passed a large amount of blood from the rectum. He became weak and clammy and his friends immediately headed the boat back to land and brought him directly to hospital. There he was diagnosed as having colon cancer and at surgery it was found that although the cancer had bled profusely, it appeared to have only infiltrated nearby pelvic tissues. The local lymph nodes appeared to be unaffected and scans suggested that the cancer had not spread to vital organs such as the liver. A section of the colon was removed and Ronan made a remarkably rapid recovery. Within four weeks he was back at work as if nothing had happened.

When he came to see me a couple of weeks later it was simply because his surgeon had suggested that he do so for follow-up monitoring. He was in great form and proud to have made such a rapid recovery. The surgeon had told him that there was a good chance that all the cancer cells had been taken away and he accepted that without question. In any case Ronan was the type of person who could put his troubles to the back of his mind and get on with life. This he was doing, and he declared that he did not have the time to be sick, so he wouldn't be troubling me too much. When I brought up the subject of *The China Study* and the association between animal protein and cancer growth he promised to read the book, but I could see that he was not in the mood to discuss it for the moment.

A couple of months later I had a report from his surgeon that all was well and that there were no signs of any recurrence of the cancer. I heard nothing more until seven months after surgery, Ronan developed jaundice. As he had been given the all-clear by his surgeon at his previous check-up he chose to come to see me. I organized a scan of his liver and this showed multiple secondary cancer deposits. To me it appeared to be a mortal blow, but Ronan shrugged and took the news with his customary good-natured stoicism. I commiserated but he smiled resignedly as he went off to see his surgeon.

There was still positivity, it seemed. Apart from the cancer Ronan's health was very good, so the surgeon decided to go for broke and remove the section of the liver where the cancer was located. This was followed by a course of chemotherapy. All that could be done had been done.

When Ronan came to see me he was under no illusion

about his situation. I quietly but firmly suggested that now would be a good time to start on the animal-protein-free diet. He had read Campbell's book but, even though he considered its assertions plausible, he told me that he was not yet quite in the mood to fully commit to the diet. He promised to cut down a little on cheese, but insisted that he would continue to eat meat. It was hardly enough, and I told him so, but I accepted the compromise, as it was better than nothing.

Ronan eventually decided to give up work completely and to devote more time to his sailing. In spite of his laid-back attitude and apparently sunny outlook he was acutely aware that someone in his position might not have very long to live. Over the next few months he remained adamant that he would not commit fully to the diet. "Life is tough enough already," was his usual response to my entreaties, and he informed me that his surgeon had not yet given up hope of curing him.

For a time no new symptoms developed and Ronan's scans remained unchanged. But just as he was becoming more confident about his future, another cancer deposit was discovered in the soft tissue of the pelvis. This was judged to be either a relapse of the original tumour or possibly a new primary lesion. It was treated first with radiotherapy, then by surgery; and this was followed up later with a further course of chemotherapy.

For Ronan this was the turning point. The sudden return of the cancer profoundly shocked him and he reviewed his options with a new seriousness. With the conviction of a man with one last chance, Ronan decided to surrender to the animal-protein-free diet. Even then we had to do a little bargaining. He loved meat in all its tasty varieties, he insisted, so while he would give up all other animal protein, he would reserve the treat of chicken for dinner once a month. Naturally, I conceded. Not my ideal scenario, given the science and the situation. But it was a breakthrough with this charmingly stubborn patient.

What ensued was nothing short of amazing.

Almost immediately after adopting the diet Ronan began to feel considerably better and after three weeks he became quite enthusiastic about his new regime. I had made a pact with myself to avoid psychological prompting and to resist coaching individuals' response to recovery. My job was merely to introduce the facts, urge the diet and to observe and record. Accordingly, I hardly commented when Ronan reported his dramatic improvement. I suspected he might attribute his new sense of well-being to the last surgery and the follow-up drug treatment he had received from his specialists, but instead he was convinced that it was the diet that had made the difference. In any case, he continued with the diet and over many months continued to feel better. A year after his last surgical intervention the oncologist took advantage of his continuing good health and gave him a further single treatment with the latest, most promising chemotherapeutic agent available, just to make sure.

Since that time no new developments have been reported by his specialists. A single very scary incident did take place, but Ronan never told them anything about it. Two years after beginning the diet he spent a month sailing with friends off the coast of France. They spent most of their time at sea and all the others on the boat were committed meat and pizza eaters. Ronan felt that he had little alternative other than to give himself a break from the diet. Two weeks after going back on animal protein, he began to pass small amounts of blood and mucus in his bowel motions. He came to see me as soon as he got home, by which time his new symptoms had been present for two weeks. We talked about his options and we both decided that if he went back on the diet and was determined to "sin" no more, the situation could be monitored at home for a fortnight. If after that time he continued to pass blood or mucus in his bowel motions, he was to report immediately to his oncologist. As it turned out, no more bleeding took place and he quickly regained his sense of well-being. It is now more than 18 months since these events unfolded. No new emergencies have emerged. Ronan appears fit, well and optimistic. He maintains a full, active life on the diet – and it looks like he has got away with it.

Melissa

Melissa was an attractive, blonde woman of 34, with a first-class honours degree in economics, when she was diagnosed with a brain tumour. This was two years before she had heard of *The China Study*. She had already undergone surgery and received chemotherapy and radiation treatments. The presenting symptoms had been headaches and episodes of distorted vision. Her doctor at the time had first thought that these symptoms might represent a form of migraine, as this condition existed in her family, but within a few weeks the symptoms had worsened and a scan confirmed the presence of a brain tumour. It had, Melissa told me, all happened so quickly. Everything in her life had been going well, she had just landed a very good job with a commercial bank and she had met a very suitable man and was in love. Now suddenly all her hopes and plans were completely shattered and she felt like a hostage to an illness she had no control over.

There was a strong history of cancer in Melissa's family. Her father had died of colon cancer in his forties and a number of aunts and uncles on both sides of her family had died of cancer at a young age. At surgery, Melissa's tumour was classified as a grade 3 anaplastic glioma. These are usually serious tumours of aggressive malignant cells that quickly infiltrate surrounding brain tissue, making it almost impossible to completely remove the tumour.

Melissa's neurosurgeon had been circumspect about her prospects while she was under his care in hospital, but as soon as she got home she had checked her prognosis on the Internet. Best predictions were that she would probably live for five or six years. The quality of those years would depend very much on how effective chemotherapy and radiation treatments turned out to be; this is the great variable in all cancer treatments. From her reading, one thing seemed certain: the remnants of the tumour that the surgeon had been unable to remove would, despite any conventional treatments, some day begin to grow again. It would continue to grow until there was no more room for it inside her head. Then she would die. This was not a prospect that was easy to live with, even for someone like Melissa, who was strong, resourceful and full of natural optimism. It horrified her that nowhere was the possibility of a cure even mentioned. The situation, in the medium term, was hopeless.

In the absence of any hope, Melissa made the decision to end the relationship with her boyfriend and, since she was not of a religious disposition, she attempted to adjust to what she called the emptiness of her new world.

Much of this happened before I'd read *The China Study.*

It was while I was in the process of considering my best approach to a study with my patients that Melissa telephoned to say that she was not well and thought that the tumour had returned. She had developed a fever and the mild headaches that she had on a continual basis since her surgery had become much more severe and were now reminiscent of the headaches she had before the cancer was first diagnosed. I detected her overwhelming anxiety and tried to reassure her. In truth, the symptoms didn't sound too serious to me but in the circumstances, and because I wanted to have some quiet time with her, I decided to visit her at home.

I examined her and was able to quickly assure her that her hour had not yet come. This time at least, she was in the clear. She was simply suffering from a viral infection. She perked, but the intense anxiety was evident in her eyes. I could see that she was struggling with understandable despondency and I was grateful that I had *The China Study* to talk about. I told her the whole story of how the book had been given to me and that while I had very little experience of using the diet with patients, Professor Campbell's and the other studies had convinced me that animal protein likely had a great deal to do with the way cancers grew. I asked her to give the diet a trial and suggested that because brain tumours do not normally metastasize the diet might be particularly effective in her case. I emphasized that if an animal-protein-free diet stopped her tumour from growing she would be cured.

I could see that Melissa was far from convinced, but I had brought a copy of *The China Study* and I handed it over. My strategy got half a smile from her. Her expectations were grim diagnosis, surgery plans and despair management – and I was giving her a paperback gift. I made her promise to prioritize reading the book, to start the diet and to phone me to let me know how she was getting on.

Melissa phoned three weeks later and I could instantly hear in her voice that she was feeling better. I offered to drop by to see her after I finished at the office.

A striking transformation had taken place. She gave me a full smile and in spite of reciting her reservations about the inconvenience of the diet it was obvious that she was in a much more positive frame of mind. She told me that she had begun to feel better within two weeks of starting the regime. She admitted that, as a discipline, it hadn't been easy. All of us are prone to comfort indulgence when we are under stress, and food "fixes" are often alluring. But she said she developed a new emotional energy once she dove in. Simply committing to the diet had made her feel that her destiny was to some extent now back in her own hands. The awful burden of despair that had plagued her since the tumour had been diagnosed was gone. More revealingly, her headaches had miraculously disappeared.

I teased her about what appeared to be effusive optimism, but it was impossible not to acknowledge the physical transformation. I examined and questioned her carefully. All her functions were normal. Her full energy had returned. She was well. I told her that in my opinion the tumour had already ceased to grow and that, with youth on her side, there was now a very good chance that her own natural defence system would kick in and finish off the job.

On subsequent visits to my office, Melissa confirmed that she was fast returning to her old self. With her improved energy levels, she had returned to work with a new sense of purpose. Whereas previously she had been driven by ambition to merely get ahead in life and to make money, there now seemed more time to devote to clients and she began to see them not just as a pile of folders on her desk but as real people whom she felt privileged to help. Her work had become far more rewarding. Another great source of satisfaction that resurfaced at this time was her love of music and of the arts. She had always been a talented pianist and a good amateur painter but as a consequence of her illness she had neglected these aspects of her life completely. With her newfound vitality, she felt drawn back to the piano and even found that her fingers possessed a lightness of touch not previously there. She took up painting again and even took on a number of young art pupils with whom to share her joy.

Every time I saw Melissa I encouraged her and congratulated her on her progress. Neither of us expressed any doubts about her future or allowed any negativity into our discussions. It could not have been going better. However, as the day of her visit to her neurosurgeon and her next MRI scan approached, I did feel a certain amount of apprehension. We had striven for positive thinking together and been rewarded with positive results. But the science had yet to be tested and, I confess, I wasn't certain yet what to expect. I felt it my duty to have a cautionary word with Melissa. But she would have none of it. At least on the surface she continued to portray utter confidence in her recovery and seemed fully convinced that the diet was working. She told me in no uncertain terms that she was looking forward to the scan as a rubber stamp of confirmation.

As it turned out, the results could hardly have been better. The tumour had reduced considerably in size and what now remained was a smaller, five-centimetre calcified mass situated in the left frontal lobe. Her immune system appeared to have walled off what remained of the tumour from the rest of the brain.

The neurosurgeon was delighted. He indicated that what remained of the tumour could probably be removed in a straightforward surgical procedure. He performed the operation a few weeks later and the histology now indicated that the tumour had changed into a low-grade astrocytoma. As far as the neurosurgeon was concerned, Melissa had been cured.

All this took place some three and a half years ago and during that time I have only seen Melissa twice. She has had the appropriate follow-up scans and all the reports show that the tumour hasn't returned. She has made an excellent recovery in every possible way and now leads a normal, happy life. There was one scare, however. A couple of incidences of rectal bleeding did occur and with her family history of colon cancer, this was a cause for concern. Could it be that after winning her battle against a brain tumour she would die of another cancer? If my theory – the one built on Professor Campbell's work – proved true, cancer cells should not grow and flourish while she was following the strict animal-protein-free diet. If they did, then my belief about the relationship between animal protein and cancer would have to be looked at again.

I'm glad to report this is not how the story evolved. Melissa had a colonoscopy and no trace of cancer was found. The cause of the bleeding was haemorrhoids, and these were easily dealt with.

Because we were all shaken by the scare and to ensure that no nasty surprises lay in store, Melissa proceeded with a full clinical check-up which involved ultrasounds, mammography, CT scans and blood tests. Happily all of these tests came back normal.

Melissa's smile had now become radiant and permanent. For me, her case reinforced my conviction that *The China Study* diet works and it increased the urgency I felt to bring news of its benefits to all cancer sufferers.

Andrew

Andrew's case proved unusual because he was introduced to *The China Study* 18 months before being diagnosed with cancer. He had suffered a heart attack when he was 60 and my reason for telling him about the book then was its sidebar claim that the diet was also efficacious in preventing coronary heart disease. This claim was based on the theory that people prone to coronary heart disease had some sort of intolerance to animal protein that could cause the lining of coronary arteries to become inflamed and lead to the deposition of plaque. A diet low in animal protein was also naturally low in cholesterol. This was a novel approach to another major global health problem – indeed one that ranks among the most stubborn and prevalent in my own country – but I had decided not to push the curative theory in the same way as I was doing with the cancer treatment approach, as it appeared to me there was at this time insufficient proof available.

I told Andrew about *The China Study* and how it had been introduced to me by our mutual friend, the geneticist, Paddy. I knew he had the highest regard for our pal, whom he had worked with for a number of years. Andrew made the decision to start the diet in the hope of preventing further episodes of his coronary heart disease. I felt encouraged, and looked forward to watching his progress.

Some 18 months after this coronary care chat, Andrew arrived at my office complaining of passing blood and a few suspicious pieces of tissue in his urine. At first, I thought this tissue might represent bits of kidney stones but as there had been no pain associated, this was far from certain. I arranged an ultrasound of the lower abdomen. This reported a "soft tissue mass" at the base of the bladder, which was a sign that Andrew had a tumour.

In the hospital tests that followed the urologist discovered a large solid tumour in Andrew's bladder. To the specialist's surprise, however, the tumour did not appear in any way aggressive and it proved possible to remove it without the need for open surgery. Unfortunately the histology showed it to be a squamous cell carcinoma and the urologist informed me that these particular tumours were among the most aggressive and dangerous of all bladder cancers. Virtually all of them carried a dismal prognosis and the standard procedure was to remove the bladder immediately to prevent the tumour from spreading. In Andrew's case there was some advantage, however. The urologist explained that he couldn't justify removing the bladder as – unusually – there was no evidence that the cancer had invaded the underlying bladder muscles. It seemed a near miss, but was clearly a puzzling, complex situation that would require careful monitoring.

Andrew's upset with the diagnosis was echoed by my disappointment. According to him, he had been on an animal-protein-free diet. If the science was right, that diet should have prevented the cancer from growing. When I discussed the matter further with Andrew, I heard his confession. The diet he promised as a countermeasure to recurrence of his coronary heart disease had been, in his words, "an on-and-off affair". I reeled a little, and re-evaluated. I read again the urologist's reports. Andrew's case had been unusual. The urologist was at pains to point out there were few, if any, cases of non-aggressive squamous cell bladder tumours in the medical literature. Why had Andrew been the exception to the rule? What was different in the course of his particular pathology?

I welcomed the consoling possibility that the diet contributed to his lucky break. Perhaps even this haphazard engagement with a new food discipline had been enough to stop the cancer becoming aggressive? Perhaps, had it not been for his diet, Andrew might have lost his bladder and perhaps his life. We talked about it. I told him of my suspicions, but he had partly made the deduction himself. A new pep talk was not needed; he just smiled, shook my hand and exited my office with a bounce in his step. He immediately resumed the diet, and has stuck to it.

Things have been going very well for Andrew. Over the past six years his bladder has been checked every three months and the urologist, who knows nothing about the diet, is beginning to believe that Andrew's may turn out to be the exceptional case that defies the normal laws of aggressive bladder cancers. Specialists go by the books, though, and Andrew's consultant still insists that the most likely outcome is that the cancer will return aggressively. The clinical monitoring continues and I carefully follow every screening report. From time to time, some of the reports I receive indicate areas of cancer in situ (non-active cancer lesions) and areas of leukoplakia. Leukoplakia is a pre-cancerous condition in which a number of surface cells undergo a certain amount of genetic change, though not enough to make the onset of cancer inevitable. In hindsight and with the benefit of observing Andrew's pattern, it seems likely that the small fragments of tissue that had passed in his urine in the first instance probably came from areas of leukoplakia. The isolation of the bladder tumour seems unique, and uniquely interesting.

Andrew receives his three-monthly lab reports with a certain amount of equanimity but, I admit, he is not yet without fear of the cancer returning. The monitoring helps his peace of mind. I, on the other hand, have become quite confident. Andrew's case remains for me an excellent example of the protective versatility of an animal-protein-free diet.

Seán

I have never met Seán but his story turned out to be such a success that it is worth recording. Some years ago a lady came to my office to see me, but instead of addressing her own minor complaints she straight away began talking about a colleague of hers whose name was Seán.

Seán had been diagnosed with cancer. That very morning, he had been informed that he might have less than a year to live. As a result, she and everybody else at work were in a state of shock. Seán was very popular, only 29 years old, handsome, active, with a reputed IQ of 150 and round-the-clock energy. The very last thing one would have suspected was that he was suffering from a life-threatening illness.

Cancer of the rectum had been diagnosed the previous year. Although this was an exceptionally young age for this type of cancer to develop, there was a strong history of the disease in the family, so when he had presented to his doctor with blood in the bowel motions, a clinical investigation was arranged immediately. It seemed that the cancer had been caught early, as at surgery no evidence was found of any spread outside the bowel itself. A small section of bowel was surgically removed and scans showed that the cancer had not spread to any other parts of the body. Seán was assured that the prognosis was good. He recovered and was back at work within two months.

Seán seemed to thrive and within a year he was making marriage plans. It was a cause of great excitement in the office as he was set to marry another staff member and everyone had been invited. However, just four weeks before the wedding day, Seán suddenly developed a nagging cough and he noticed with alarm that there was a trace of blood in the sputum. His doctor was not overly concerned but a chest X-ray was carried out for caution. To everybody's amazed horror, multiple cancer lesions were found in both lungs. A biopsy confirmed that these were secondary deposits and that the cancer had come from the original site in the colon. Seán was devastated and asked his surgeon whether it was advisable to go ahead with his marriage plans. The surgeon was obliged to lay it on the line: the fact that this was a secondary cancer with the lesions in both lungs meant the prognosis was very uncertain. It would be best to postpone the wedding.

This information about his new diagnosis was just in. Little wonder that, on the evening of the day he had cancelled his wedding and informed his work colleagues of his situation, my patient spent most of her session talking about him rather than herself. She wasn't looking for miracle answers, but she was clearly a woman of some empathy. She felt bad for Seán and was reaching for some words, however tenuous, of hope. The case sounded so advanced and irreversible that I hesitated to propose *The China Study*, or to discuss the informal trials I had in hand. Seán was not my patient. On the other hand, the extremity of the case and the poignancy of Seán's situation called for some positive effort. I told her about *The China Study* and suggested that she give Seán the book. He had youth on his side – and a youthful immune system. If Professor Campbell's logic was correct, a quick switch to the animal-protein-free diet might – just might – stop the cancer growing. I didn't want to upset any apple carts, but I told my patient to convey my best wishes to Seán and to tell him he could telephone me at any time if he wished.

As it happened, I heard from neither of them during the next six months. To be honest, I was disappointed. I blamed myself for failing to engage sufficiently and with enough enthusiasm at the time. But when I examined my conscience, I knew that the truth was that I believed his case was too far advanced. Professor Campbell's work suggested the likelihood of extraordinary cancer treatment results when a specific countermeasure was rigorously applied. It was no miracle agent.

I had almost forgotten the whole incident when, out of the blue, I received a text message from my patient. It read, "Simply have to tell you about my young friend with the cancer in his lungs. Recent scan shows NO growth in the tumours! He gets married tomorrow. In view of the fact of no growth, chemotherapy has again been postponed at least until after his next scan. Doc was amazed. We thank you for *The China Study.*"

Some months later my patient phoned to bring me up to date. Seán had apparently immersed himself in the diet after reading Campbell's book and had made such a dramatic recovery that he amazed himself, his fiancée and the doctors. The improvement in his health was such that, with the specialist's blessing, he had decided to go ahead with the wedding. He was back at work full time and had avoided chemotherapy as his symptoms improved. The lesions on the most recent scan were smaller, though they had not disappeared completely. Today, she told me proudly, he felt well and was symptom free.

In the ensuing months, I had intermittent text messages from my informant keeping me up to date with what was going on. No further growth of the cancer deposits in the lungs took place but, on the specialist's advice, another chemotherapy session was given for safety. This appeared to have had the effect of lessening the size of the lesions but – again – not eradicating them. What was most important was that Seán continued to be symptom free. It wasn't just my patient and I who were rejoicing in this development. Seán's case was apparently remarkable enough for his specialist team to have opted to present it at a major medical conference. I investigated this and was crestfallen to see that the case was put forward as a curiosity rather than anything else. His consultants saw Seán's progress as an example of how bizarre things sometimes happen with cancer. The animal-protein-free diet was mentioned only in passing and not discussed in any detail by the medical professionals at the conference.

It is unlikely that any of the attendees came away believing that eliminating animal protein had an important role to play in stopping Seán's cancer. While I found this heartbreaking, I was encouraged to remember that it was merely by reading *The China Study* that Seán found the conviction to try a diet that might be worthwhile. For me, this case was a restorative.

If, simply by reading a casebook of results, one sufferer could be helped to outfox his illness, so others could. "But supposing Seán's survival *wasn't* down to the diet alone?" one cynical friend chided me. "Chemotherapy has undisputed therapeutic value." I don't doubt it, I told him. But it's only a diet, for heaven's sake. Be cynical. Sidestep the evidence before you. Forget that it works. But at least take it to the great medical institutions for dedicated, *focused* application and study. Neither doctors nor patients have anything to lose by doing so.

Michael

Michael's story provides more evidence of the sensitive relationship that exists between animal protein and cancer. When Michael was 30 years old he suddenly began to complain of headaches and episodes in which his vision became blurred. Neither symptom was very marked but it was worrying all the same. A brain scan was performed which identified a large, frontal tumour, and the biopsy revealed that the tumour was a low-grade, mixed oligoastrocytoma. As these tumours are usually slow-growing and do not normally metastasize, complete removal can often result in a cure, but because in this instance the tumour had already infiltrated a part of the brain associated with vision, surgery was not an option for Michael. It was decided therefore not to offer any invasive treatment for the time being but to simply monitor the situation and await the onset of more severe symptoms before taking action.

Three months later Michael developed epileptic seizures. These attacks consisted of violent jerking movements of the arms and legs, loss of consciousness and often biting of the tongue. Generally they lasted for a few minutes but each attack was followed by confusion and drowsiness that sometimes lasted an hour or more. The seizures were terrifying for Michael as they also were for everyone witnessing them. Anti-epileptic medication worked well for a time but the dosage of the drugs had to be consistently increased to maintain relief. Eventually the drugs ceased to be effective altogether and a decision was made to try "debulking" surgery. The aim of this was to take away as much of the bulk of the tumour as possible without damaging the surrounding brain tissue. In this way it was hoped to decrease the pressure of the tumour on the areas of the brain that were causing the seizures to occur.

The debulking surgery did no more than modify the seizures and lessen their frequency. As the situation remained progressive it was decided to see if a course of radiotherapy would help, and with the combined effect of the anti-epileptic medication, the debulking surgery and the radiotherapy it finally became possible to put an end to the grand-mal-type seizures that were so frightening for Michael and his family. Unfortunately, after a few more months these seizures were replaced by the much milder petit-mal attacks. These seizures consisted of brief "absences" during which Michael's mind would suddenly go blank and for a minute or so he would be completely unaware of where he was or what was going on around him. Onlookers would hardly notice that an attack was taking place, but nonetheless these muted attacks became crippling. They were so frequent and debilitating that they prevented him leading any sort of a normal life. He could not be left unattended. The unpredictable frequency meant that he had to be accompanied whenever he was away from his home. This, of course, had a dramatic effect on his freedom and the quality of his life. As a result of the new rules, he spent a great deal of time confined to the house, watching television and eating. His specialist team suggested the prognosis was just a few years' survival.

At this point I was actively looking for volunteers to participate in my informal trial. When Michael came to see me with his father for one of his regular check-ups, I immediately told him about *The China Study* and suggested he should try going on the diet. My suggestion was met with derisory laughter from both Michael and his father. The very idea that he would have to stop eating meat, cheese and pizzas was ludicrous as these were his culinary staples. Prior to his illness, I was reminded, he was a very fit, large-framed football enthusiast. He had especially enjoyed the customary inebriants and gustatory indulgences that post-match socializing in the local pubs mandated. These activities had already been seriously curtailed because of his tumour and the seizures. Was I was really asking him to sacrifice yet more? Undeterred, I tried to talk up the culinary possibilities of an animal-protein-free diet. The look on his father's face said I was wasting my time but I knew how much Michael dreaded the epileptic attacks and I persevered. After much arm-wrestling we finally managed to strike a deal. Michael would go on the diet for one month. If all seizures did not stop within that period he could go back to his beloved steaks and pizzas.

Much to my delight, it worked. Once Michael gave up animal protein, the attacks lessened in severity and all epileptic seizures stopped completely after just three weeks. I have to be honest – I did not expect such a dramatic result. At best I had hoped for a gradual diminution in the number of seizures and I had planned to renegotiate the diet deal with Michael on the strength of that.

On his father's advice Michael went along to see his neurologist to tell him about our encounter and its apparent result. Fortunately the neurologist put forward no objection to the diet, though he firmly opined that it was unlikely to have played a role in the cessation of the seizures. In the specialist's view, Michael should remain on the medications that most likely caused the attacks to stop. He patiently explained that with brain tumours it was not unusual for seizures to come and go. When Michael came back to see me to report his talk with the specialist, I didn't dispute the advice he was given. But I did suggest that, since it was an indisputable fact that the seizures had ceased, it would be foolish to stop either his medications *or* the diet. When he hemmed and hawed, reminding me how much he loved his pizzas, I reminded him that we had made a bargain.

For two years Michael had no epileptic attacks and consequently I saw him less and less. I received regular reports from his specialist team that his scans were satisfactory and I heard from his father that he was finally doing some part-time work and getting back to many of the activities that had been part of his former, normal lifestyle. He had become a regular at the gym once more and was determined to regain his athletic physique. During all this time he apparently remained faithful to his diet.

Some months of silence passed and then events moved rapidly – but not in the right direction.

When next I heard from his father, I learned that Michael was back socializing again at full force. He was travelling, attending football matches and enjoying all the usual post match revelry with his friends. When I probed, I was told he had gone back to drinking substantial quantities of alcohol and eating large steaks. His revised version of the diet decreed that he could eat whatever he liked when not at home. He told his father that he wasn't prepared to commit to the animal-protein-free diet anymore. He was fixed, he said. And that was the end of it.

Within a few weeks I was saddened to hear his condition had suddenly deteriorated and that the headaches and frequent seizures had returned. When his father brought him to see me I was heartbroken that our alliance was gone. He was no longer interested in the diet and didn't want to listen to me. Life is too hard, he said, to suffer sacrifices. The comfort of tasty food of every variety is too seductive.

Shortly after our sad session a scan was carried out that showed the tumour had grown again. Further debulking surgery was undertaken and a biopsy showed that the tumour had now transformed into an aggressive anaplastic glioblastoma. Post surgery Michael received chemotherapy and radiation treatments, but these were unsuccessful in arresting a rapidly worsening condition. Personality changes occurred and Michael developed weakness of his left arm and leg and lost the sight in one eye. His brain was obviously damaged beyond repair and he slipped into unconsciousness and, in a matter of days, died.

5

The Specialist Stumbling Block

"It is dangerous to be right in matters on which the established authorities are wrong."

– VOLTAIRE

DOUBTS AND HESITATIONS

The main obstacle to patients given the diet on trial is the fact that no support has been forthcoming from the cancer specialists. When patients mention the fact that they are considering the diet to their specialist they are routinely told that they are wasting their time. More often than not, they are reminded that animal protein supplements are regularly used to help patients recover from the ravages of cancer and the side effects of chemotherapy or radiation treatments. The only nutritional advice generally given is that patients should eat well so as to keep up their strength to fight the cancer. All too often at the first sign of weight loss, the suggestion is made by oncologists that protein supplements should be added to the diet. There is no account taken by these specialists of the fact that such supplements are mostly made from dairy produce and therefore are more likely to feed the cancer than to help the patient's recovery.

In an effort to prepare the patient for the specialists' antipathy towards the diet, I generally forewarn them that they are likely to face discouragement and so perhaps it is best not to tell oncologists that they are on the diet. I know this is a ruse, but I also ask them to bear in mind that cancer experts are unlikely to know much about nutrition and I reassure them that an animal-protein-free diet will not interfere in any way with the standard treatments they are likely to receive. The result is that most of the patients who read *The China Study* and commit to the diet do not inform oncologists that they are doing so. This predicament, paradoxical as it sounds, suits my purposes. As the general practitioner who is the patient's intermediary, I assume in the eyes of the specialists a neutral stance. Consequently, instead of derision and evasion from cancer departments, I tend to receive more detailed reports on how the treatments are progressing and the full results of the various scans and tests. In my experience patients are happy enough to go along with this little bit of deception and the advantages are obvious. Having full access to the details of how the patients are progressing is essential to my research. I encourage my patients to accept whatever treatments are suggested by their specialists and I can best interpret the effects of the diet, at least in the short term, by comparing the progress made while on the diet with the results I would have expected to see had they not been on the diet. This may appear to some as far too subjective a manner to make accurate judgements. But after 40 years in medicine, experience dictates expectation. Given the conventional surgery-radiotherapy-drug approach, in the normal course I would have expected the majority of my patients taking part in the trial to be dead or at least at an advanced stage of their disease after prolonged treatment. From the start my study has shown this is not the case and this exceptional indicator demands, in my mind, the fullest possible inquiry and evaluation.

Most people are not aware of the very powerful hierarchical system that exists within medicine. They routinely encounter the front line – the local GP – and assume there is a joined-up service ranging from pharmacy providers to the most esteemed consultants, all closely linked and ready to interact with his or her needs. This, sadly, is not the case. The process of diagnosis and treatment is a fragmented area in which, at present, specialist medicine rules the roost. This is not meant in any way to deride the brilliant, dedicated laboratory and trial work done in specialized clinics all over the world. But communication *is* a bugbear. Each specialty is regarded as the sole repository for all available knowledge on a particular subject and, as a consequence, any advances can only come from *within* a particular field of specialty.

Herein is the rub. Whereas, unquestionably, new ideas and new theories on how best to tackle cancers are constantly surfacing, they are debated in the specialist journals where peer review deems their appropriateness (or otherwise) for further research investment. These results then finally filter down to the less specialized medical journals and, ultimately, to the GP and the general public. This I believe to be a system that is inherently flawed because it blocks or fatally delays progressive ideas from those outside the given specialty. It seems a tragic irony that the idiosyncratic bias of the specialist might be indulged and funded, but the ideas contained in, say, *The China Study* simply cannot qualify for explorative *inclusive* discourse.

The inception of specialized medicine can be traced

back to René Descartes, who established the philosophical framework that gave birth to the model of the specialized medicine that exists today. A French-born mathematician and philosopher, Descartes firmly believed that human beings could best be understood if they were regarded as being assembled in much the same way as a machine. He suggested that all of the mysteries of the human body could be solved by the reasoning power of the mind, and he was responsible for a mechanistic line of thought in which all parts of the body would be linked up intelligibly and be made understandable to all. In his writings about physics, Descartes proposed "to divide each difficulty into as many parts as is feasible and necessary to resolve it". This reductionist concept provided the template for specialist medicine and directly led to its formal establishment. Through the process of dividing the body into its individual functioning units, one could see how each function worked and thus better understand the workings of the whole. Reductionism quickly demonstrated how the different systems of the body are interdependent and how a disease in one system can lead to the destruction of the whole. This new insight heralded many triumphs in the evolution of modern medicine. As a consequence, the human body was peered at as never before. Every magnification of the microscope was applied to all structures, and new findings of interrelation dispelled long-held erroneous beliefs pretty much overnight. These objective scientific methods provided the hard facts that medicine had previously lacked and made past theories seem naive.

Once all the anatomical details required by a particular specialty had been established, efforts were made to understand everything about how the physiology of that part of the body worked. Among other things, this usually involved analysing the chemical make-up of a particular system of the body and attempting to understand what sort of catalytic processes could affect it. Once the normal levels were established, medical scientists could then focus on determining which changes were taking place in the particular system when a person was suffering from a disease. This was a form of reverse engineering that eventually led doctors to establish a methodology for diagnosis based on reviewing the body's chemistry. If one looks at the enormous amount of information that now comes from X-rays, EKGs and cutting-edge scan technologies, one begins to appreciate the influence that Descartes' reductionism had on modern medicine.

With such a wealth of knowledge it became inevitable that more and more fields of specialization would be defined. Reductionism led to a virtual atomizing of the patient. Medicine became an area of exponential growth, inevitably leading to new methods of treatment and a vast range of new medications. When, in 1928, Alexander Fleming discovered penicillin, its stunning efficacy as a treatment for infection won over the world. In the age of rapid-growth media, the general public was educated on the effectiveness of medication. People of the era had lived through the 1918–20 flu pandemic which had killed as many as 100 million people, one-fifth of the world's population, most through secondary infection. No persuasive treatments were available then; now, suddenly, mankind could fight back. For medical science, the floodgates opened. In the next few decades there were medications developed to treat depression, control blood pressure, kill pathogenic microorganisms, destroy cancer cells, relieve asthma, lower cholesterol and alleviate pain.

Whereas doctors of an earlier age relied on herbal remedies, bloodletting and chance, now there was an artillery of thousands of drugs and combinations of drugs with which they could fight illness and improve their patients' prospects.

The consequences of all social advances, whether cultural, economic or scientific, must always be carefully weighed. History has taught us that there is often a downside. In the case of medicine, the advances in diagnosis, treatment and drug development meant that mechanical man thrived in the twentieth and twenty-first centuries. As new forms of communication shrank the world and our standard of living improved, death statistics also radically improved. By the end of the twentieth century, for example, the infant mortality rate in the Western world had declined by more than 90 per cent, and maternal mortality rates had declined by almost 99 per cent to less than 0.1 reported deaths per 1,000 live births. Modern man and woman, cosseted by science and clinical medicine, were living to a ripe old age. The corollary, of course, was a new challenge to medical services in light of an increased – and increasingly aged – population developing new diseases and geriatric complications. The response, one would think, should have been the streamlining of health services, based on the modern advantages of instant communication, genome-level research and a holistic interweaving of all we have learned in the centuries since Descartes. In fact, this is not the current status quo.

The governing principles remain correct. The medical profession and the pharmaceutical industry have become partners in the war against disease. I have no dispute with this. The specialist community, armed to the teeth with the most up-to-date medications, have become the generals conducting the battles. I have no dispute with this, either. But one could question whether the interests of the patients, the doctors and the chemical companies always fully coincide. "Holism", as we have seen, is medicine's defining byword. Its dictionary definition is "intimate interconnection, such as they cannot exist without the whole." My argument about the current status quo – and the challenge posed by the emerging facts about nutrition I was encountering now in my everyday experience – is an issue of holistic medicine, discovery and communication.

The first results of my informal trial convinced me that the sort of dietary manipulation suggested in *The China Study* worked in combating, even conquering, cancer. And I saw an excitement among many in my patient group when this awareness dawned on them. But I also saw a kind of muted helplessness, because they were sorely aware, too, of the gap that existed between my surgery and the specialist rooms they attended. I meditated long and hard on how to tackle that gap. It was daunting to consider the potential outcome if the medical community adopted a comprehensively different approach to nutrition management. How would the dents in medicine's relationship with the pharmaceutical companies be mended? How would the oligarchs of supermarket food chains respond to changes in retail policy?

The status quo – today's standards – is fundamentally unchanged from the *status quo ante*, yesterday's standards. Money rules. It is foundational in state building, in everything. This story reaches a point of confession: the challenge of my own sense of inadequacy. As I've said, my early survey perfectly reflected the results of Colin Campbell's meticulous animal-protein studies. I saw the truth of it, living and breathing in my own suburban surgery. But I confess that my scheme to record and report it swooped to a grim nadir when I contemplated the monolith we were facing. Forget status quo. Cynicism, fed by vested interests, would drown us, I was sure.

And then I thought about Descartes and the courageous whimsy that inspired his most important work. Today he is regarded as the father of philosophy, the father of analytic geometry, the father of rationalism. His *Meditations on First Philosophy* continues to be a standard text at most university philosophy departments and his work is required reading around the world for third-level students of mathematics. But all this great work began with a moment of profound retreat. In November 1619, while stationed as a military engineer in Neuburg an der Donau in Germany, Descartes locked himself in what he called an oven room, to meditate. He sat up all night and later wrote that he experienced three visions during his contemplation. He saw a chain of order simply subdivided. Science, he sensed, would be the path of true wisdom for him. In wisdom would be learned that all truths are interlinked. And then, circularly, one fundamental truth would lead by logic to an understanding of all science and existence. *Cogito ergo sum* – I think, therefore I am – was the genius summation that arose from this abstract, radical thought experiment, and its cogency sparked an intellectual renaissance that gave modern man the confidence to take better control of his own environment.

The lesson to be learned from this is, perhaps, the value of isolation. Thinking outside the box is self-explanatory: you need to absent yourself from a situation to objectively address and resolve it. I've always enjoyed reading about the outsiders like William Blake, H. G. Wells, Van Gogh, Kafka, T. S. Eliot, Beckett, T. E. Lawrence, Gurdjieff and Dostoyevsky, who subtly reoriented society's values.

All espoused revolutionary ideas and were opposed and derided along the way. They suffered the slings but they were not deterred. What all had in common was a persistent determination to be heard. And a devotion to hard work.

I wavered, but I went on.

6
Standing Alone

"Nothing strengthens authority so much as silence."
– LEONARDO DA VINCI

PUSHING AGAINST A CLOSED DOOR

I was by now utterly convinced that there was a genuine case against the safety of a diet containing animal protein for those affected by cancer, and this compelled me. In my mind I could see Paddy the geneticist smiling at me. He knew me too well. He knew I was a stubborn devil likely to brave out the first stumbling block, the scepticism of my colleagues. The fact that none of them showed the slightest interest in the relationship between diet and cancer was not a deterrent. The second stumbling block, the institutional "wall", was a little trickier. Collusion with my patients was the Trojan Horse, and a sense of solidarity drove me onwards. Still, a sense of propriety, the ghost of the age-old Hippocratic oath, made me constantly check myself. Was my stubbornness doing the best service to my patients? Was my process beneficial to the medical profession?

I was repeatedly drawn back to beginnings. It was Colin

Campbell's influence, and his particular courage, that had set me on my way. I thought more about him, and about the boundaries society sets for us and those we set for ourselves. Theoretically, we are all free. We are blessed with free will and can make of the world what we will. We have choices and can carve out for ourselves the life we want. But of course reality is more contingent than that. We live in an unpredictable world moulded by material vicissitudes and by stubborn social patterns. Civilization commands structured community sharing and all such structure-building mandates a hierarchical order. The consensus has chosen the model of the world we live in and the institutions we have created to keep our civilization sound are inviolable, or at least corralled by the laws that protect them. Institutional medicine stands stoutly at the top of a mountain. Generally we accept its dictates and submit to it in silence. But what makes someone take on the entire medical profession? Professor Campbell, a nutritionist, had certainly stuck his nose into a subject that medicine deemed none of his business. It took something beyond a long-shot theory and fortitude to conduct the experiments, write the book and risk the institutional wrath as he had done. Reading about his childhood on a dairy farm, where he learned the importance of personal responsibility from an early age, provided some insight into the character of this tenacious man. Perhaps he and I had something in common? Inherent self-reliance was something we surely shared. In his case it dated back to the unending duties of farm maintenance. For me it was my time as skipper of a lobster boat.

I had an uncle who lived on Achill Island, off the west coast of Ireland. He was a businessman and the owner of some trawlers and small motorboats. When I was 12 years old, I asked him if I could borrow one of his boats for the summer months. The plan was to make a little money by supplying lobsters to the local hotels. From about the age of nine I had spent much of my summer holidays going out on the boats with his workers. I do not know how he rationalized his decision to allow a 12-year-old to take sole charge of a 35-foot motorboat, but when I asked for the boat he only raised an eyebrow and said, "Well, okay." I was doubly surprised because I had fully expected to be scorned. Looking back on it, I can only conclude that he saw something in me that I did not know I had. The only knowledge I had of what it took to run a vessel was that I had gained from watching the experts who operated his fleet. I was bright, so my uncle probably guessed I'd learned the essentials about navigation, and more importantly about engines, just from watching them. That was a huge assumption. The truth was that I had no idea of how an internal combustion engine worked. I knew how to turn a key or pull a traction cord. I knew that when an engine wouldn't start, the men usually scraped the plugs with a knife, and if this failed to do the job, the next trick was to suck or blow out dirt from the pipe that fed the fuel to the engine. That was my graduate thesis.

In any event, it was enough for my uncle. He shook my hand and the deal was sealed. He gave me 30 lobster pots and wished me luck. In today's world he would probably have been locked up, but it was a vote of confidence in me that I never forgot. For about four summers my 11-year-old friend Aodán and I worked as lobster fishermen. We had no lifejackets, mobile phones, flares or any means of communicating with shore. From early morning until dusk, in the often very rough seas off Achill, we baited the pots, set them, lifted them and sold our catch to the hotels. I was the skipper but as Aodán knew more about fishing than I did, he did most of the directing. I only asserted my skipper status when the sea got rough and we were in danger of going onto the rocks. We never did make a great deal of money, but they were great, character-building years and I believe that what happened during those summers prepared me for practically everything else that has happened in my life since. I learned that it is impossible to live without risk, but that risk management is everything. I learned the values of breaking ranks and standing alone. More than anything I learned in those summers that the courage to make decisions is the most liberating form of bravery.

STANDING ALONE IN ALABAMA

I am going to recount some of my adventures in Alabama as it may help you to understand why an ageing doctor like me would take up a nutrition expert's baton and become evangelistic about so critical an area of health care reform.

Our characters are indeed moulded by the influence of our parents, our religious upbringing and our cultural inheritance, but it is often chance happenings that endow the streaks of individuality. I believe that becoming the skipper of a lobster boat at the tender age of 12 moulded essential aspects of my character; it certainly led to my seeking out independence in my life earlier than most. I was drawn to medicine for its nobility, by the fact that it gave individuals the opportunity to help people and, perhaps in small ways, lessen the burdens of life. Shortly after graduating in 1960 I sought employment as a junior doctor at Mobile General Hospital, in Alabama. I know my family expected me to find work more locally. But the same impulse that sent me into lobster fishing, sent me to Alabama. Be under no illusions;

this was hardly the sort of position that was likely to further my career in medicine, but the words "Mobile, Alabama" resonated. I knew nothing about the Southern States beyond a schoolboy awareness of the legacy of the Civil War and what I extrapolated from reading *Gone With The Wind.* But I was drawn by intuition to a place of challenge.

The freedom to work anywhere in the world was one of the great advantages of being a doctor. My father, who was a psychiatrist, had used this argument in persuading me to study medicine as an alternative to lobster fishing. He fully understood my sense of daring and I'm glad he encouraged me. So it was with a great sense of freedom that I set off for the US on one of those very large Cunard liners that dominated the Atlantic in days of yore. I was 24 years old and without a care in the world. I chose to cling to the romance of it all. After years of deskbound study, this was my first long-overdue truly adult adventure. It took six days to make the crossing to New York City, just about the right length of time to allow one to pack away all memories of childhood and prepare oneself for the unknown. At six o'clock in the morning the ship berthed and I was up on the deck amid a crush of passengers as we slipped past the Statue of Liberty. As I looked at the misty-eyed faces of my fellow passengers gazing at the Manhattan skyline glistening in the early morning sun, I knew how meaningful this moment was. For the Irish, this was the promised land, the land of freedom and hope. As a young adult I felt privileged to be starting my career here, not just because of the enduring link of sentiment and history that binds our nations, but because America was consolidating its position as a visionary place, a place of science and democracy, where shortly its youngest ever president, the Irish American Jack Kennedy, would be pledging that the nation would to go to the moon by the end of the decade, thus opening untold floodgates of new knowledge and opportunity.

The aeroplane due to transport this young Irishman to Alabama was scheduled to leave the following morning, which meant that I had one full day in which to explore the fabled New York City. I took a yellow cab to the hostel where I'd booked in for the night and, having deposited my bags, set off wandering the extraordinary canyons of Manhattan. Television and movies had given me notions, but nothing prepared me for the futuristic dynamism of Manhattan's grid. Skyscraper after skyscraper, hotels, churches, banks and department stores, all disgorging crowds who bumped and jostled the occasional wanderer such as me. The sun got hotter and hotter as the morning wore on and I was suddenly sweat-drenched in my Irish woollen suit. I spotted a gents' tailor shop and went in. When the salesman heard I was bound for Mobile he suggested I try an off-the-rail cream linen suit with light navy stripes. "Just right for Mobile," he declared triumphantly, and even though I felt it more suited a vaudeville stage, I conceded and bought it. I left the store transformed, a Southern gent if ever there was one.

My first day in Mobile is emblazoned on my mind. From the moment I stepped off the plane every pore of my body gushed sweat. Now I understood the Manhattan salesman's subtle nudging. The heat and the humidity were far greater than anything I had ever experienced, but it wasn't disagreeable. This was after all the Deep South, and I think I would have been disappointed had it been anything less. A surly African American took my bags and put them in the limousine that was to take me to my final destination. He looked at the label and smiled. "You're the very first white

Kelly I ever seen." He had a soft, warm drawl. I presumed he was kidding me, but I preferred to think he was serious.

I relished that half-hour drive from the airport into a new life. Magnolias were in blossom, every house was made of wood, there were sprinklers on every lawn and a kind mist enveloped everything. In my naivety I thought it was a fairyland. When we stopped in front of 750 St Anthony Street, the driver gestured with his hand and said, "Here we are." I looked up and down the street. Mobile General Hospital did not look like a hospital at all. It had the façade of an old colonial house with a balcony that ran the whole length of the building, looking down on the street. All it lacked, I felt, was a Stetson'd frock-coated gent with his boots on the rail, chewing tobacco and chatting up some decorous ladies with frilled parasols.

Once I passed the Palladian columns, though, the illusion was dispelled. This was a spic-and-span modern hospital, as clean-floored, functional and purpose-designed as anything I had known in Ireland or Britain. I was impressed.

I was shown to my room in the front part of the building behind the old colonial façade. This room was journey's end and was to be my home for the next year. What most struck me was how cold it was. Air conditioning was something we'd never had in Ireland and I didn't care much for the chilly dryness of the air. I hurried to open the glass doors that led to the balcony, and when I did a blanket of humid heat immediately swept into the room, enveloping everything. Already I had come to delight in American warmth and I knew I would be at home in hot, sticky Mobile. Sitting down on the wrought-iron rocking chair on the balcony, my feet comfortably propped on the elegant little wrought-iron table, I surveyed America passing by on the street below, with a sense of smug fulfilment. This, I thought, is going to be a breeze.

Complacency is an unhealthy state of mind. Though my work was due to start the following day, I hardly gave it a thought. Alabama, I reckoned, was something of a medical backwater and I'd surely, effortlessly, hold my own here. Then I found a little booklet in the room with information about the hospital and the staff. I immediately saw I'd been naive in my assumptions. Four members of the staff had trained at the celebrated Harvard Medical School, which, even as far away as in Ireland, was renowned and respected. So much for my smugness. Perhaps I was not quite the medical "catch" for Mobile General that I thought I was. Suddenly the room was hotter than comfortable and I was closing the window to bolster myself with that cool, reviving air conditioning.

Mobile General in fact turned out to be quite a surprise and taught me an early lesson about doing the research. Unbeknownst to me it had a reputation of being an excellent teaching facility and its association with the esteemed Birmingham Medical School elevated its status. The hospital was well managed and most of the doctors on staff turned out to be wonderful teachers. Unlike many I had come across in the past, these doctors enjoyed teaching. Here I learned what the phrase "American know-how" really meant. Everything was modular and strategic. Firstly I was taught all the practical techniques I would need for my work around the hospital. Individual doctors taught the skills they themselves possessed and then personally supervised the newcomer until they were assured that the techniques had been mastered. It was a kind of jigsaw approach. By the end of my year in Mobile I could deliver babies, do minor surgery, deal with accident cases and manage every conceivable medical emergency that was ever likely to befall a person. Those skills taught in Mobile General have stood me well over the years and I have always been profoundly grateful to the doctors for their commitment.

Beyond the hospital walls, though, Mobile was undergoing tectonic cultural changes. I'm ashamed to say I was unfamiliar with its racial dilemma. I understood the outcome of the Civil War, of course, and knew that the Southern States had passed contentious legislation in the early twentieth century to disenfranchise African Americans by creating barriers to voter registration. I knew, too, that Alabama's ever-increasing population, boosted past the 100,000 mark by the wartime shipbuilding boom, was substantially black. But I had heard that huge progress in civil rights had been made, the Jim Crow laws were being eroded and such institutions as the local police force and Mobile's celebrated Jesuit Spring Hill College were fully integrated. Once again, complacency. I was giving the newly elected Kennedy and the Democrats too much credit for a new fairness in government and was about to discover that "my Alabama" was a selfish fantasy.

Over time, I observed that nobody wanted to discuss the racial issue. The practice of boycotting segregated institutions was sweeping the South but at the hospital, staff – and patients – seemed more interested in the status of the Pittsburgh Pirates versus the New York Yankees. All members of the staff, coloured and white, appeared to get on very well together. One would never have known a social problem existed except for the fact that the cafeteria was divided into separate seating areas and the drinking-water fountains in the corridors were always in twos, placed a few feet apart and labelled "White" and "Colored Only". Reflexively, I think, I turned a blind eye. In my Irish innocence the situation seemed, at worst, quaint – though in hindsight I think I was psychologically blanking out reality in hopes of maintaining my idyllic image of the place. I fastidiously did my work, kept an eye on progress towards the World Series and learned to drink my water elsewhere.

For the first six weeks all went very smoothly at Mobile General. Then an incident took place that almost cost me my job. I had been assigned to a surgeon for the first part of my rotating internship and I was assisting him in removing the appendix of an 18-year-old black girl. The surgeon was a mild-mannered middle-aged man and we had been getting along very well together. He was a terrific teacher and, as usual, on this particular day he was talking away, showing me how to perform various procedures in the process of the appendectomy. The operation went well and just as he was finishing he stopped talking medicine and began telling me about how well the Alabama State football team was doing that year. I listened interestedly to the football talk but just as he was getting ready to close the incision, I suddenly saw him put his finger into the wound and loop out a fallopian tube. I presumed he was checking to see if the tubes were healthy but then I realized he had a different agenda. When I casually asked what he was doing, he raised his eyebrows and looked somewhat severely at me. "I'm going to tie her tubes," he said. "You know all these girls have too many babies." There were no coloured nurses in attendance at the operation and I could see that everybody in the operating room was looking expectantly at me.

This was unprecedented, beyond anything I could ever have imagined in medical care. The frozen moment was like an incident of high drama in a Wild West movie, with me grimly in the leading role.

"Does she know that you're doing this?" I asked, my mouth a little dry.

The surgeon shook his head.

"Then I can't let you do it," I said.

There was a terrible wall-like silence. Visions of instant dismissal, an ostracized life, a roughing-up or worse from the fabled Ku Klux Klan all came flooding into my head. The surgeon looked at me with a gentle smile and shrugged. He did not even seem annoyed as he said, "Okay, I won't if you don't want me to."

He closed the wound and I took off my surgical gloves. I did not know what my next lines in the movie should be but I had the awful feeling that the camera was still on me. "I feel obliged to say I will have to report you to the hospital manager," I stammered.

The surgeon shrugged again, but as I left the operating theatre there was an ominous atmosphere and nobody was smiling.

I went straight to the manager's office on the top floor, fighting a nauseous tension. I had never met the supervising manager, but as I entered his rooms I felt sure my days at Mobile General were numbered.

The manager turned out to be a very affable, bald-headed man in his mid-forties. He smiled a welcome and shook my hand warmly as I introduced myself. I told him what had happened in the operating theatre and he sat back in his chair, nodding. He was neither angry nor surprised and I could see that he understood the predicament I found myself in. He spoke quietly: "Yes, a few of them do that, I'm afraid. They know that I don't approve, naturally, but they do it anyway."

He seemed to think those words were enough, but of course they would never be. I cleared my throat and told him

I would have to report the incident to the American Medical Association.

He snapped to attention, shaking his head firmly and frowning at me like a disappointed father. "I wouldn't do that," he said. "You have no proof of what happened. No one who was present will corroborate what you are claiming, and the surgeon would never admit to it. Remember that."

The manager watched me carefully for several minutes as I wrestled with these appalling facts. Then he smiled benignly. "Look, give me a few days and I will see what I can do," he said. "Don't talk to anyone about this." He shook my hand, and I left his office, utterly crestfallen.

I did not have a restful night. The personal implications induced anxiety, but the moral issue was completely depressing. Was this the reality of institutional medicine? What I had been taught in Dublin about standards was based on the highest ethical and moral values. That was the foundation on which the science was based. Was I now to be forced to recalibrate my thinking? Were there geographic aspects to medical ethics that I hadn't accounted for? Would I find that morality was a variable, that what was accepted in one domain was invalid in another? A double standard, I decided, was out of the question. My spontaneous impassioned complaint might have rocked the boat, but I was glad I showed my mettle. Institutional reinterpretation of morality wasn't, I concluded, acceptable on any account. My knee-jerk response was appropriate, let the cards fall where they may.

Two days later I met the surgeon who had performed the appendectomy, in the hospital corridor. He and several fellow surgeons had talked about the matter and had decided to desist from performing further unrequested sterilizations.

"I reckon it was going a bit too far," he admitted. The apology was watered down to a political excuse: "I suppose we risk giving the hospital a bad name, so you were right."

I decided to let the matter drop. The battle, if not the war, was won and within the hospital, culturally, the point had been made. The fact that I was promptly assigned to another surgeon for the rest of my time in Mobile didn't bother me. That first surgeon had taught me invaluable lessons about the evolving American society, about the necessity for alert responsibility in *all* areas of patient care – and about myself.

Lobster boat skippering established my contentment to be an outsider and gave me my focus and my grit. To be most effective within the medical community, I learned in Alabama, these attributes would be invaluable.

For all of us, remembering our beginnings has the potential to serve us well. One must always embrace fate, but one must equally be prepared to tackle its vagaries. In Alabama, perhaps, I was prepared to confront convention in some future, dramatic way.

Alabama showed me how small actions can have huge impact. I reminded myself of that as I dove back into my determined scheme to get *The China Study* a proper, fair hearing.

7

A Revolution of Thought

"A little rebellion now and then is a good thing."
– THOMAS JEFFERSON

Persuading patients suffering from cancer to eliminate animal protein from their food intake is especially problematic in Western countries, where dairy and meat are very much part of our daily diet. Constant, clever, all-media marketing makes the benign cow, the pig and the lamb popular culinary choices. Add to this a reassuring slice of science: the proteins contained in these animals' make-up are almost identical to those found in the human body. So it seems logical to suppose that consuming animal products is the very best course for humans and is ideal for nourishing and repairing the body's cells. For humans the fact that our favourite food is also the favourite food of cancer cells doesn't compute. There is a psychological block, which I believe is nothing less than tragic.

We are all aware that meat and dairy produce have come under suspicion in recent times. During the last decades of the twentieth century, well-funded, coordinated and transparent research showed these foods were implicated in coronary heart disease, which, along with cancer, accounts for most premature deaths worldwide. It was the meat and dairy fats, and in particular the cholesterol, that were shown to be the problem. At the time it was difficult for people to accept that the foods they had been reared on since infancy might be associated in any way with fatal disease. Yet when the scientific medical community banded together and produced their irrefutable results, the doctors cooperated in encouraging people to accept the findings, and the pharmaceutical industry – and indeed the food industry – made the appropriate adjustments to promote and produce anti-cholesterol drugs and foods.

The difference between that situation and the role of animal protein in cancer is one of focus. For the coronary heart risk, *unified* research took place. The Seven Countries Study that formally started in the autumn of 1958 in Yugoslavia and engaged four regions of the world – the US, Northern Europe, Southern Europe and Japan – is still ongoing. It has carefully compiled its findings with well-disseminated, coordinated recommendations and, after 50 years, is still well-funded and continues to fine-tune the results. By contrast the targeted research to support the indications that animal protein has a major role to play in human cancer is still fragmented within generic "nutrition" studies. Much of the problem may lie in as-yet-undiscussed global economic fallout. Medical institutions – whether the World Health Organization or the most futurist start-up labs – are dependent on either government funding or private benefactors. Governments have a vested interest in economic stability: the food industry, as it has been honed for centuries, is an inviolable, economically sound model. Private benefactors are often wealthy investors whose altruism is combined with investment savvy: pharmaceutical profits are legendarily huge and consistent. The cash support that comes from both these sectors is the lifeblood of clinical studies. What government will invest heavily in trials that prove its principal food-trading ethos is unsafe? What investor or pharmaceutical industry chief, benefiting hugely from the proliferation of cancer drugs, will invest in studies that might lead to the demise of much cancer drug production? Should a link be verified between animal protein and cancer growth, clinical procedures would change so fundamentally as to command food producers to completely remodel their product and their methodology; it would also close door after door to drug producers. Oncologists might also find their services comprehensively reordered as their expertise in drug administration and management becomes downgraded. Such a quantum shift in the recognition of the aetiology and treatment of cancer would obviously be economically, even nationally, disruptive. It might have a deleterious effect on the livelihoods of many, and would certainly lead to institutional and procedural changes at the highest level. These considerations give cause for pause, but they cannot be an obstacle to truth. If science shows a definite connection between animal food consumption and cancer – as science tardily showed a definite connection between cigarette-smoking and cancer – the consequences must be faced, countered and overcome. National interests must come second to human interests.

In my Dublin surgery I encouraged awareness of Colin Campbell's work without overburdening patients with politics or statistics. I was encouraged by a few high-profile forward-thinkers like Bill Clinton, who publicly espoused the essence of Campbell's findings after his own health crisis. It has often struck me that popular media figures have a great advantage in airing radical views. Bob Geldof's heroic highlighting of the plight of Africa is a case in point. We all knew of the wealth disparity in the world. Oxfam recently published figures showing that 85 individuals own approximately half the world's wealth. We see the injustice, we see Africa's suffering – but it takes the loud centre-staging of a pop figure like Geldof to push our conscience into committed response. There were many times in my surgery when I wished a Geldof would come through my door. But the world I occupied was couched in the quiet desperation of seriously ill people seeking solace and the reassurance that their doctors knew best.

The dilemma created by the gap between the local GP and the specialist always kept me on my toes. I fully acknowledge the vital role specialization plays in dealing with illness, because every pathology has its own evolutionary parameters, and time and study is needed to manage the vast amount of information targeted treatments require. But there is an anomaly at work, I believe. There is a vast difference between respecting the sensible departmentalizing of specialization and handing over to specialists the unchallenged right to completely run the show. In the field of highly specialized medicine as it exists today, it is all too easy for a patient to land in the hands of the wrong specialist.

My friend Bob is an example of this. A year or so ago when I was away on leave, Bob developed symptoms suggestive of a stroke (cerebrovascular accident). He had been to the gym that morning and upon returning home had felt completely exhausted, so much so that he had to retire to bed. Suddenly, his speech became slurred and one side of his mouth became paralyzed and drooped. Bob was immediately brought to the hospital emergency room and was seen by a stroke specialist who conducted scans and other investigations. These showed no sign of haemorrhage nor any evidence of clots in the brain. All of the symptoms of apparent stroke resolved over a period of about an hour and a diagnosis of a TIA, commonly called a mini stroke, was made.

The stroke specialist was, however, not entirely satisfied with the diagnosis. Having questioned Bob carefully it emerged that the patient had experienced a number of similar, though less severe, episodes in the past and had recovered fully from them.

The stroke specialist therefore decided to solicit the opinion of a neurologist. This neurologist was an eminent doctor and his special area was epilepsy. Tests were done and although no convincing evidence of epilepsy was discovered, a diagnosis of polymorphic epilepsy was made. Bob was put on anti-epileptic medication and discharged with instructions that he would not be permitted to drive a car for at least a year and that he must stay on medication for the rest of his life. This was a pretty disastrous diagnosis for Bob, since not being able to drive would affect his work as well as his social life and would clearly limit his activities generally.

When I heard about the diagnosis upon returning from vacation, my reaction was one of surprise. I had known Bob as a patient for a long time and I was already aware of these episodes. I had diagnosed them as migraine manifestations a long time previously. There was a pattern to Bob's "mini strokes". They always came on after he had been to the gym and they always resolved within an hour. I knew him to be something of a keep-fit fanatic and he had the habit of frequently exercising to the point of complete exhaustion. Often after a session in the gym he would have to crawl into his bed for an hour's rest and sometimes the exhaustion would be accompanied by a headache. I had advised him that his symptoms were likely the manifestation of a type of migraine and that he should cut back a little on his exercise regime, as he risked provoking a stroke if he pushed himself too far.

Given the medical history and Bob's recent crisis, I felt the diagnosis of epilepsy was a shot in the dark. I told Bob I would seek a second opinion from another neurologist, this time one whose special interest was not epilepsy.

This second specialist met Bob and scanned and tested him rigorously. His findings both delighted and troubled me. The specialist agreed with me about the migraine-related indication and immediately took Bob off his anti-epilepsy medication and advised him to resume driving and resume a sensible fitness program and a normal work and family lifestyle. Thereafter, Bob thrived.

The moral of the story is that specialists can become so focused on their own particular expertise that they sometimes fail to see where the truth lies. I believe this short-focus factor is what obstructed worldwide cancer treatment progress following Professor Campbell's revelations about the dangers of an animal-protein diet. The minds of cancer specialists were so cluttered with their pharmaceutical and surgical obligations that they were unable to accommodate critical revisionary thinking. I must not be too hard on my esteemed colleagues: it is undeniable that down through the years many unsubstantiated claims have been made about the association between cancers and one food stuff or another. But the key here is substantiation. Idealistic New

Agers might *believe* a particular food causes disease, because of anecdotal evidence; Colin Campbell had *proven* the link between animal protein and cancer cell growth.

"How can you guarantee me this animal research of Campbell's will translate to my own cancer?" was a question I heard many times in my surgery.

"I cannot," was my invariable answer. But, as time moved on and patients came and recorded their feelings and progress and I had the advantage of comparison exercises, the statistical realities told their own story.

Peter

Peter was 63 years old when he developed cancer of the prostate. He had been an infrequent patient of mine over the years, but as he lived close by I knew him well. For some months he had been getting up more frequently at night to urinate. This had not worried him unduly as he simply put it down to the fact that he was getting older. However, when the urge to urinate began to interfere with his long walks and golfing, and when he began to complain of a nagging pain in the lower part of his spine, he finally came to see me. I examined him and came to the conclusion that he might be suffering from cancer of the prostate. Within a few days, the diagnosis was more or less established as a PSA (prostate specific antigen) blood test came up with a reading of more than 150. A normal reading is less than four.

Up to this point in his life Peter had enjoyed excellent health. He had a good job and he was happily married with three adult children. When I mentioned the possibility that he might have cancer it was as if his whole world came crashing down. He was devastated by the prospect and full of regret for having ignored those early symptoms. I managed to get him an urgent appointment with a urologist and an MRI scan was quickly arranged, which confirmed that cancer of the prostate was indeed present and that the tumour had already breached the capsule of the gland and had invaded the surrounding tissues. Secondary deposits of cancer were found to be present in nearby lymph nodes and there was also an area of early bone metastasis in the sacral area.

Based on this evidence the urologist telephoned me to say that the cancer was almost certainly very aggressive, and as it had already spread to several locations neither surgery nor radiation treatments were immediate options. He volunteered the opinion that even with treatment, Peter's life expectancy would probably be less than 18 months.

Although I had already intimated to Peter that there was a possibility of cancer, I had softened the blow by explaining how prostate cancer was often slow in its progression and that modern treatments were increasingly successful. He was not at all prepared for the very frank discussion that he had with his urologist. When he came to see me some days later he had already relinquished any hope of a favourable outcome. I took the opportunity of telling him about *The China Study* and explained that Professor Campbell's claims were supported by solid scientific research. He was prepared to grasp at any straw and within three days he had read *The China Study* and decided to go on the diet. When I saw him two weeks later he was utterly convinced, his deep pessimism had evaporated and he claimed to feel that his cancer had already stopped growing.

The urologist wanted him to have a biopsy of the prostate as soon as possible so that an official staging of the disease could take place, but as it turned out Peter had a number of important social and work commitments to attend to and these tests had to be postponed for a few weeks. In the ordinary course of events this should hardly have mattered, as the MRI scan had already conclusively shown the cancer to be aggressive, and a biopsy and staging of the disease would only serve to confirm this.

Peter was troubled by having to postpone the test but I put a positive spin on it. The delay, I told him, would serve as an opportunity to evaluate the potential early results of the meat-and-dairy-free diet. He huffed and puffed but agreed and seemed reassured.

His confidence, and mine, was rewarded. A few weeks later a very surprised urologist informed us both that the results of the biopsy showed the cancer to be of an intermediate grade only. The report specified that Peter's condition was "far better than one would normally expect in an untreated cancer that had already metastasized".

Peter was delighted and told me these results reflected exactly the sense of well-being he had experienced since starting the diet. Simply, he felt better. The urologist – who knew nothing about the diet – was also encouraged, but he did not alter his opinion of the overall prognosis. He prescribed a hormone treatment for Peter that I was to administer every three months. And so, with fingers crossed, we commenced. A further PSA test, taken some six weeks after this treatment began, showed results within the normal range. Always cautious, I told Peter that much of the credit for this improvement might be down to the hormone injections. I found myself in the ironic position of fielding his disagreement. It wasn't the injections, he insisted. He felt certain the diet was responsible. The physical change he'd felt since beginning the diet was too significant, he said. Day by day he could *feel* the effect it was having on his body.

One thing was certain: I could hardly have found a more persuasive advocate for *The China Study* diet. From the depths of despair Peter had become increasingly confident about his future and within a matter of weeks had returned to all his normal activities. He went from strength to strength and I now only saw him when he came to have his hormone injection. On these occasions, I highlighted the importance of continuing the diet, although there was never any doubt in my mind that I was preaching to the converted. An MRI scan performed six months after the injections had begun showed that the prostate was still enlarged, but there were no longer any signs of the invasiveness of the cancer and most of the secondary deposits in the glands and bone had either disappeared completely or become considerably smaller. A PSA at this stage gave a reading of less than two.

Peter's specialist was delighted at what he took to be a particularly good response to the hormonal treatments. Peter himself was feeling very well, but although his PSA tests remained in the lower range of normal, the mass of the tumour remained large and continued to cause obstruction to the flow of urine. The urologist had hoped that the tumour would get smaller in time but this didn't happen. Eventually, in order to relieve the symptoms of excessive frequency, two years after the diagnosis of cancer was first made, a decision was taken to remove part of the tumour surgically. While the surgery succeeded in its primary aim of relieving the obstruction and thus the symptoms of urinary frequency, some months after this a scan showed multiple bone metastases. This did not come as any great surprise to me and probably not to the urologist. Of course

I support surgical intervention when it is required, but I have reservations about its efficacy in certain circumstances. While removing a tumour entirely can sometimes cure cancer, I tend to believe cutting away a part of the tumour can risk cancer cells entering the blood stream and allowing them to set up secondary deposits in other areas of the body.

It seemed to me that the prognosis had drastically changed. Peter commenced a course of chemotherapy that he tolerated reasonably well. I was disheartened but I told him we still had artillery in our alternative arsenal. If he stayed on his diet, I felt, he had the potential to prevent the secondary deposits from growing.

And this appears to be the outcome. Peter has regained his vitality and is once again confident about the future. A CT scan performed four months after the secondary deposits were found in the bone showed "no evidence of disease recurrence".

I received the specialist's report yesterday.

Patrick

Patrick's story is included not because his cancer was particularly dramatic, but because it serves to illustrate how the cancer of patients who have responded positively to an animal-protein-free diet may quickly revert to an active state if the diet is not maintained.

Patrick was undergoing investigations for symptoms of bladder outflow obstruction when a superficial bladder cancer was incidentally discovered. The cancer was removed straight away and the histology report showed it to be a grade 3 papillary transitional cell tumour with lamina propria invasion. There were also areas of carcinoma in situ (non-active cancer) present. The urologist told him that, although there was little immediate danger, he would require regular three-monthly check-ups since this sort of situation could easily turn into aggressive bladder cancer if left untreated.

Although obviously upset by the diagnosis, Patrick was nevertheless reassured that his life was not in any immediate danger, and when he came to see me some weeks later he had more or less come to terms with his situation. I told him about *The China Study* and suggested that by going on an animal-protein-free diet it should be possible to ensure that the cancer never became aggressive. The detailed science in the book sufficiently convinced him to make the necessary changes to his diet, and in all of his subsequent check-ups over the next couple of years there was never any sign of active cancer. Occasionally areas of carcinoma in situ in the bladder were reported, but Patrick was reassured that because such cells are inactive they can easily be treated, and hence there was no cause for concern.

Patrick duly became more and more confident and even began to suspect that the urologist had exaggerated the severity of his original condition. His increasing confidence did not cause him to stop attending his specialist, but it did have the result of making him a little careless with his diet. Avoiding all animal protein had never been a great hardship for Patrick as he had grown to like the wide range of foods permitted. But he did report a social problem. His job entailed entertaining clients at city restaurants several times a week. Most of these clients were meat eaters, he said, and not all restaurants he went to had varied non-meat menus. The discipline of sticking to an animal-protein-free-diet had become irksome. Under his own steam Patrick reread *The*

China Study and decided that he had been applying its rules too strictly. He established a new agenda for himself that would allow him to suspend his diet when eating out with clients.

Within a few months Patrick was in trouble. At his next regular check-up a few small areas of early invasive cancer were discovered alongside the carcinoma-in-situ lesions. Patrick's urologist carefully explained that the in-situ cells, which had undergone genetic change, were now actively multiplying. This, he said, wasn't a surprise; it was just proof that the three-monthly check-ups were necessary so that new areas of activity could be dealt with and tackled.

For Patrick, however, the news was a sobering experience. He blamed the situation on the laxity that had crept into his adherence to the diet. There were too many parallels, he told me, between the progression of his illness and his moderated animal-protein intake. I agreed with him. In the course of watching many patients adopt the diet I had seen this correlation often. I told Patrick so, and I emphasized to him that deviating from the diet meant the cancer could return, but I believed he had the remedy in his own hands.

What is most instructive about Patrick's case is the clarity of correlation. For almost three years we stayed in close touch and he stuck to the diet religiously. The cancer abated and he was in excellent health. Then, sadly, complacency set in. The distraction of normal life prompted him to start eating steaks and traditional breakfast fry-ups. In no time the cancer returned actively and vigorously. I was appalled but I wasn't surprised. What was happening to Patrick was an exact replication of the laboratory responses Campbell had observed in rats, where the levels of animal protein in their diets dictated the expression or abeyance of cancer.

Patrick had kept his carcinoma-in-situ areas in check while he was on the diet. Once he reintroduced animal protein, the foodstuff of cancer cells, he kick-started malignant cellular activity.

At the time of writing, Patrick has begun a course of treatment under the direction of his urologist, in which BCG vaccine is injected in the bladder in an attempt to destroy all carcinoma-in-situ areas that might so far be unseen. My own view of the case, based on my informal trial, leads me to believe that this is unnecessary, as Patrick has now fully committed to diet-controlled cancer management and is stubborn about his intent. He has seen the risk in lapsing and believes that dedication to the diet removes the threat of any aggressive cancer reappearing.

Let me emphasize here that my hardened belief, arising from cases like Patrick's, is no pat response. As already stated, I possess the natural conservatism and calculation of my professional training. Even as I embarked on my trial, my belief often wavered and it did not easily become a conviction. But as results piled up, self-persuasion was no longer an issue. For 40 years I had seen so many cancer patients in my surgery who followed the orthodox treatments suddenly take a turn for the worse and die. Only with the animal-protein-free diet did I see a fight back. Cases like Patrick's presented the clarity of a barometer. Faithful to the diet, they improved. Faltering, their cancers became aggressive. After every such encounter my faith in the essential wisdom of *The China Study* increased.

Beyond faith is fact. What most inspired me in cases like Patrick's was the immediacy of remedial results. Many, many patients reported very early on that the diet was having an unarguably beneficial effect. Many experienced a dramatic improvement in their sense of well-being after just weeks. As intelligent, objective people they were naturally astounded by the turnaround in their condition. Their positive feedback encouraged me to continue with my research and it fortified my ambition to see the medical profession take on the responsibility to unify resources in researching the implications of Colin Campbell's breakthrough study.

8

Passing the Baton

"Man cannot discover new oceans unless he has the courage to lose sight of the shore."

– André Gide

SYNCHRONICITY

About half way through writing this book, I received a most unexpected affirmation of my belief in the validity of my clinical work with the diet. One morning, as I was spending time fiddling around with sentences and trying to make the words I had written sound more persuasive, something curious happened. During a short break from writing I had turned on the radio as a distraction. I wasn't making any particular effort to listen to the discussion taking place, nor did I know who was speaking. Then, in a moment of reverie I suddenly heard the most unlikely and most gratifying words: "the effect of some proteins on cell division". They had an almost electrifying effect upon me and I hurried from my chair to turn up the volume. What I had stumbled upon was an interview with a British biochemist, Sir Richard "Tim" Hunt, and he was being interviewed on the occasion of his retirement from The British Research Institute. It was a moment of curious synchronicity.

I listened attentively to the discussion and it soon became clear that unbeknownst to me a considerable amount of research had been taking place in biochemistry for a long time on the subject of the effect of certain proteins on cell division and replication. This research was being undertaken on both sides of the Atlantic and the radio presenter recounted how in 1982 Tim Hunt had made some of his most outstanding discoveries when experimenting with sea urchin eggs at the Marine Biological Laboratory at Woods Hole, Massachusetts. His most important discovery was the identification of two specific proteins, cyclin and CDK, which are instrumental in ensuring that cell division takes place in an orderly and controlled fashion. In fact, his findings were so monumental that he was awarded the Nobel Prize in 2001. It was encouraging to hear such a revered scientist talk about a causal relationship between proteins and cell replication, because this interactive relationship was the core of the dietary theory espoused by Colin Campbell, based on his own research program.

Bizarrely, just a few weeks after hearing the Tim Hunt interview, another moment of serendipity occurred, suggesting further corroboration. I was glancing at the magazine section of the *Financial Times* when I came across an article on another well-known scientist. It was an interview with James Watson, the geneticist who, with Francis Crick, had famously discovered DNA in 1953. He too had been carrying out research into proteins. Although in his eighties, Watson was continuing his work at Cold Spring Harbor Laboratory in the USA. The research project he was now involved in was attempting to discover gene-activating protein inhibitors (RNAs) associated with specific cancers, so that, once identified, their action on cellular development could be blocked.

In the interview Watson explained how a newly discovered gene-activating protein called bromodomain-4 had been found to be essential for uncontrolled cell division to take place. In his view there was now a very real hope that within the next five to ten years a broad-spectrum chemotherapeutic agent would become available that was likely to be highly effective against a large number of different cancers.

It is not necessary to grasp the finer details of these new discoveries to immediately appreciate the corroborative link between such research and Professor Campbell's theories on the dangers of animal protein. Hunt and Watson were separately proving that individual proteins had a marked effect on the manner in which cells divide and replicate; Campbell had demonstrated that the elimination of all animal protein from a diet given to cancer subjects blocks unhealthy cell development. The correlation is too specific to be overlooked and my stumbling on these parallel research studies fortified my commitment to my trials.

A word here must be said about synchronicity, the concept of meaningful coincidences that are unlikely to be causally related, first introduced by Carl Jung in the 1920s and finally published in 1952 in a volume with a related study by Nobel laureate Wolfgang Pauli. For Jung (and the intellectuals who later took up his cause, like Arthur Koestler) life was not a series of random events, but rather an expression of a deeper, revelatory order. Rolling, 24-hour news and the unregulated information deluge of the Internet tend to taint any new knowledge with a militant scepticism. This reflex isn't new, of course. In medieval times visionaries like Copernicus and

Galileo were castigated for their breakthroughs in science. The common accusation levelled at cognitive scientists is the alleged problem of "confirmation bias", that is, a tendency to search for or interpret new information in a way that confirms one's personal preconceptions. Apophenia, a related aspect of so-called critical thinking, finds patterns in nature where none exist: the face of the man in the moon, for instance. But the synchronous aspects of my experience scientifically contests the weakness in the paradigm of contemporary critical thinking. Colin Campbell started with an observational theory that indicated animal protein might be problematic in our diet. His careful, empirical lab studies bore out this theory. My observations of patients' life patterns and personal instinct set me on my own course study. But I was not actively seeking new strata of scientific corroboration. I found it extraordinary – and indeed very welcome – that Hunt and Watson came knocking unbidden.

What all of this meant for me was that, instead of the isolated feeling of ploughing a lonely furrow, I had the sense of working in a like-minded, if disconnected, global team, all of us nudging forward and finding validation for our work in confluent results. I have to admit that discovering Hunt and Watson felt like moments of epiphany. Unquestionably big names and much-awarded authorities have the capacity to make all the difference in any ideological movement. James Watson said it is "a virtual certainty" that the work now being carried out in his laboratory will result in new cancer drugs being developed. These words alone filled me with optimism and renewed vigour. The road we were on – my trial patients and I – was a valuable one and may take us across a threshold that none of us can yet fully evaluate in terms of the improvement in human life.

Fear of change, however, is a mountain to be reckoned with. As fate would have it, a very personable exchange with a medical specialist a short time later reminded me of the gap between the labs of Campbell, Hunt and Watson and the common lives of GPs and their suffering patients.

We'd met at a social event held in a hotel in the southern part of Ireland. He was the son of an old friend of mine and I had known him since he was a young boy. He had gone on to become a very distinguished professor of gastroenterology working in a Dublin hospital and had acquired a reputation as a first-class medical teacher. The old family friendship meant that when he spotted me at the reception, he immediately crossed the crowded floor to greet me. We had met very rarely over the years but the warmth of his greeting was as it had always been. On this occasion he had a distinctly wry grin on his face and he asked me straight out how I was getting along with my theories on animal protein. It was evident that his father had informed him about my trials, and I could see from his demeanour that, just like his father, he reckoned I was barking up the wrong tree.

Because I was in the middle of compiling this text, I welcomed the opportunity for intelligent discourse to help gather my thoughts. What better subject to bounce ideas off than a worthy, esteemed member of the medical profession? I recounted in detail the essence of *The China Study* (by now so embedded in my mind that I could recite it in my sleep), and then gave him a careful, dispassionate account of how my more successful diet-controlled cancer cases were faring. I knew most specialists wouldn't have bothered listening. In the age of arrogant science, the age of affluent torpor, the age of television cynicism, I could take my place in the queue with Copernicus, Jung and Koestler. Within a very short space of time I saw that the young professor just didn't want to hear any more.

I knew what was coming as he held up his hands to shut me up so he could begin his diatribe.

"Have you any idea of how many patient cases you would need to undertake and how much documentation you would need to amass in order to have even the remotest chance of being taken seriously by the profession?" he said. "John, your research is not even remotely scientific. Where is your peer review? At the very least you would need other doctors to back your views, and from what I have heard so far, I doubt very much whether such backing will be forthcoming. You need to stand back from your fixation on animal protein and consider the possibility that you may be wrong! At the moment all you are doing is simply pushing a totally unproven dietary cure for cancer, seemingly oblivious to the fact that there are already hundreds of similar cures out there. You have to remember that there are thousands of research professionals busily at work all over the world, researching every possible cure for cancer. Do you claim to know more than anybody else? Who do you think you are? Are you perhaps The Chosen One that everybody will automatically listen to?"

He was animated and spoke passionately, but there was no animosity. He seemed amused by me and I wasn't at all offended. In fact, I almost applauded. I smiled warmly, feeling a sense of gratification. "I needed you to tell me that," I said. "It clears up any doubt that I might have had about the problem of the specialist community."

"You mean people like me?" he grinned.

"Yes, you really are all the same. Because you are so

accustomed to being the acknowledged experts, pontificating comes naturally to you. You only know the texts of your own rule books. You find it impossible to consider subjects outside the remit of your own small area of expertise. You are trained in such a way so that once you are outside your comfort zone you must immediately pass the issue at hand to some other 'expert' who professes himself a specialist in that separate field. But the trouble with the animal-protein problem is that no such expert exists in your elite club, and as a consequence the problem remains improperly examined and unresolved."

I didn't stop there. My young friend sat smiling as I trotted out my hobbyhorses one by one: the long history of uninventive medicine that allowed such indulgences as bloodletting; compartmentalized over-specialization that turns patients into isolated guinea pigs; the fact that much medical research is compromised in principle by the funding that comes from multinational drug companies; the bullying of a vision of global political democracy based squarely and solely on economic concerns. I was amused by myself. To the casual observer I might be Noam Chomsky preaching social anarchism. "All we ever hear about in contemporary psychology and social policy is the value of critical thinking. The so-called 'well-justified conclusion' must be meticulously sought. But those in positions of strength and power have an obligation to investigate new and alternative studies. This, for their own vested reasons, be it complacency or fear, is not pursued. The well-justified rationale is just a sound bite. Professor Campbell's very reasonable theory has not been researched properly in globally coordinated human studies, in my belief, because of a mixture of institutional self-interest and stubborn backward-looking prejudice. My dilemma is moral conscience. I have read and checked *The China Study* and I believe it to be vital as a foundation for reassessing cancer treatment. But neither you nor your peers will listen because I am not in the specialist club. I have been left in a quandary. I could ignore the implications of Campbell's work for my fellow man, or act on them. I am acting, in my surgery trials. So what your peer community has done is to obligate me to carry out research that you and your specialist friends are more suited to. You sarcastically suggest I might be The Chosen One. If I am, it is because *you* have chosen me. It's a lazy option for you, because you and your specialist colleagues are not prepared to do the work."

His "Wow!" was followed by laughter. "I don't know if I deserved all that, but perhaps it will do me some good. 'We' don't get spoken to like that very often. Although there may be validity in some of your points, I still say the theory of an association between animal protein and cancer is far-fetched."

"Why?"

He chose to divert. We were, after all, friends. And this was just social banter, its fundamental seriousness notwithstanding. He patted my arm affectionately. "As for my remark about you being The Chosen One, John," he said, "I regret that phrase. It seems to have gone to your head!"

Our exchange had done us both good. A table for two became vacant just beside where we'd been standing and fortuitously a tray of drinks passed and we grabbed two glasses and sat down. He was right: the moniker of The Chosen One had gone to my head. It's not that I'd absorbed it in any religious sense, but it triggered some reflective thinking. Spontaneously I found myself musing on the strange serendipitous things that have happened over my lifetime. It was suddenly pleasing to have an amiable professorial colleague to engage with, if only to parry and provide some devil's advocacy.

"Since we've risen to spiritual matters, let's talk about destiny," I began, and from his smile I could see he was up to the challenge. "I'd like to hear your views on that," I said. I saw him stalling, his eyes fixed calmly on me while the cogs and counters of evaluation spun. Was I teasing him? Surely I wasn't about to take him down that New Age road of evangelic whimsy, the road dotted with stores selling positive-thinking cure-all adages on cheap greeting cards? Should I reassure him of my educational earnestness? Of my fidelity to the rules of my training? Where would we start? The moment when psychology separated from medicine, or psychiatry from philosophy? Psychiatry as part of holistic diagnosis? The subdivisions of psychiatry, as defined by the separation of the therapeutic techniques of Freud and Jung? Theosophy stretching beyond the wars of religion to find the lost wisdom – Aldous Huxley's *Perennial Philosophy* – that may realign communal spiritual thinking? I had carefully read and assessed it all and come to the opinion that no era owns truth. The religious rules of the early Christian years are not the Christian rules of today. The science of the Pharaohs is not the science of MIT or CERN. But each era yields visionaries and breakthrough moments of confluence and harmony from which the future is built. One must forever be cautious and questioning, but scepticism as our current culture has it is just cynicism in a fancy dress. And cynicism, in my view, is valueless. I remember smiling inwardly, and somewhat sadly, when I read the famous quote of Adlai Stevenson, the American Democratic contender in the 1952 election, when he was told that Norman Vincent Peale, the motivational writer famous for *The Power of Positive Thinking,* opined that Stevenson would make a poor president. "I find Paul appealing, but Peale appalling" was Stevenson's response. I have my own gripes with Peale's take-no-prisoners optimism, but Stevenson's reaction seemed to sum up the ridiculous polarization of cultural thinking. Stevenson's adherence to St Paul, the principal interpreter and popularizer of the books of the Christian Bible, is no more Olympian a viewpoint than Peale's. The perspective of ever-changing history tells us there are lasting values from the oddest opinions in some of the least likely moments. We must never cease to mine the past in order to build a secure future.

"I suppose you're going to tell me you believe in destiny," my young friend said.

He hit a sensitive nerve. As the son of a psychiatrist I have always been interested in the workings of the mind and, consequently, the mind-body correlation. I was fortunate to be born in the century when the foundational breakthroughs of Freud and Jung were brought to new levels of understanding by such movements as Albert Ellis' cognitive therapy, Eric Berne's transactional analysis and Abraham Maslow's humanistic psychology, all programmes designed to enhance the individual human experience. All of these paradigms sought to embrace *spiritual* health and to explore the underlying order in existence, what Jung called the *unus mundus*, the one world, which is so often hidden from us. Jung and many other forward-thinkers believed there are signs and symbols of unifying nature all around us, potential healers who are knocking to try to gain access. Jung strongly believed in synchronicity and a universal design. While I don't particularly believe in predestination, I do believe we are born with certain potentialities and that chance happenings can cause these to either flourish or remain dormant. This I decided to share with my friend.

I was beaming a wry smile when I said, "The fact that you are sitting here listening to me may mean that you are about to discover that you have been repressing an important part of your own nature for years and maybe you are just about to wake up and change. Think about it: a little girl born into a musical house will almost certainly find herself learning how to play a musical instrument. But a chance meeting with a teacher of mathematics could suddenly bring her to a very different calling. In your case let us imagine that destiny has so far caused you to become a professor of specialized medicine – but maybe you are about to discover that there's more to you than that."

I was teasing, of course. But I sensed a value in pushing the boundary. I had encountered stubborn rejection in my attempt to arouse wider professional medical interest in Colin Campbell's work. Perhaps a new tack would breach the fence.

"My hidden qualities?" the young professor mocked.

"No one knows everything," I reminded him, "the corollary of which, of course, is we all inherit the obligation to keep learning. I'm amused when you label me The Chosen One because, who knows, there may be truth in it."

"You're joking of course."

"Semantics," I said. "Word play. But let's tease it out. Strange things happen to everyone and they're usually put down to simple quirks of fate. But I'm going to tell you some true stories about myself that may lead you to believe you might not be far off the mark in calling me 'chosen'."

I watched him mentally recalibrate. Suddenly it seemed we were characters in a narrative by Dan Brown, arrogant and incredulous by turns, sipping good wine in elegant surroundings and speculating on adventures that might grow from the most modest beginnings to change everything.

THE QUEEN OF CLUBS

"I hope you realize you are now beginning to sound seriously weird," the professor said. "I will listen, but your stories had better be good."

We both smiled as I commenced.

"This isn't about Chosen One nonsense or strange powers," I said. "There was nothing unusual about me as a child, but in my early thirties I suddenly encountered a strangely intuitive side to my nature. I call it my 'queen of clubs' experience.

"I was in the West of Ireland for the Christmas vacation with my wife and three young children. We had rented a cottage in County Clare and my brother-in-law from France had rented another cottage alongside ours for his family. A 23-year-old cousin of my wife who was studying for the priesthood in France was also staying with us. In all, there were five adults and seven children in our group. The weather that Christmas was unusually good, with clear blue skies by day and starlit nights with hoar frost. It was indeed Christmas-card weather, ideal for long walks by day and sipping hot whiskeys in the evening in front of a blazing peat fire.

"On the evening when my strange incident took place, we were chatting around the table in our cottage having just finished a game of cards. The talk had drifted to superstition, ghost tales and other strange happenings, a not unusual agenda in the West of Ireland at Christmastime. As there was no particularly gifted storyteller among us, the ghost stories fell a bit flat and, in any event, the clerical student informed us that he didn't particularly like tales of the paranormal. In his fervently religious family background, ghosts were not spoken about. Most of the group then left the table to prepare dinner, leaving the clerical student and me alone."

I glanced at my professor friend and saw his intrigued gaze. All Irish folk like a good yarn and he nodded eagerly for me to continue.

"The clerical student's reaction surprised me. I had forgotten how some religious people can overreact to talk of the paranormal. I apologized and explained to him that in Ireland it was traditional to tell ghost stories at Christmas. Where he came from, he said, all strange happenings involving the dead were associated with satanic practices and were accordingly best avoided. I was happy to leave it at that, but the student felt compelled to explain himself further. Anything ghostly, he insisted, was ungodly. As for magic, that was all down to trickery and sleight of hand. He was so adamant – aggressively adamant – that I felt the petulant urge to challenge him. I liked stories of strange events, whether the polished yarns of M. R. James and Sheridan Le Fanu or just plain old folklore, I said. They amused me, and kept me on my toes about all we don't understand and the wonders of our existence. This didn't appease our friend and he grunted disapproval. I persisted – taunting him a little, I'm ashamed to say – and I asked had he personally ever experienced an odd event in his life. Telepathy, for instance. When he frowned bewilderment I told him honestly that in my practice as a doctor it often seemed part of the normal day's work. Many of my patients related stories of their own intuitive experiences and, for myself, there had been many occasions when thoughts of a patient that suddenly came into my head foreshadowed their unexpected arrival in my office. The clerical student of course immediately dismissed this as irrelevant coincidence."

My friend the young professor nodded vigorously and said he was on the side of the student.

"Of course you are. That's why I'm telling you this story. In any case, prompted by the whiskey maybe, I searched in my mind for a way to prove my point to the student. Perhaps, I thought, I could demonstrate telepathy?"

"Ah, so you're one of the gullible ones," my professor said with a sad nod. "You believe all this charlatan claptrap."

"I know about charlatans," I said. "But I was trying to show the value of an open mind. I've read up on these issues. I understand that telepathy has been studied since the middle nineteenth century, when the Society for Psychical Research was set up in Britain. I understand that the National Research Council in the States wrapped up its own study, doing no better than to state that telepathy contradicts the laws of theoretical physics. But that was before the proposed laws of the new physics – all the quantum-based theories arising from discoveries about dark matter, dark energy and dark flow in the universe that you read about in the science section of the newspapers just about every day now."

"Meaning?"

"Everything changes. Knowledge itself is in flux. So one cannot exclude speculative theories about any phenomena, even if they are tagged with old-chestnut labels like 'paranormal'. The laws behind these things might be very normal indeed."

"Okay, go back to the Christmas ghost stories."

"I was in a playful mindset, remember. A deck of cards lay on the table where we'd been playing and I spread them out face down in a large semi-circle in front of the student. I told him I would demonstrate telepathy with the deck, but since he was such a doubting Thomas, I wouldn't touch the cards. I would be the passive observer and he would do 'the trick'.

"I asked him to pick up the cards to ensure there was nothing unusual about the deck. I then asked him to shuffle them again and spread them out himself. He did as I asked. I then requested he pick any card and place it face down in front of him. Without looking I immediately told him that the card he had chosen was the queen of clubs. I have to emphasize that I was acting playfully and spontaneously. There was no expectation of 'proof'. I was having fun. It didn't matter to me one way or the other what the outcome was, but I did ask what his reaction would be if that card turned out to be the queen of clubs. He thought for a moment and then said that of course he would immediately think I'd conned him in some way.

"This made me think again and focus a little more. I said, 'All right, let's make it harder for me. Put the card you have selected back in the pack and shuffle the deck again.' He did as requested and I told him to pick another random card. 'So what will this one be?' he asked smugly. I shrugged. I suppose it must still be the queen of clubs, I said.

"There followed a strange moment. I was in a completely neutral, even indifferent, frame of mind, enjoying the banter, the whiskey and the Christmas warmth of the fire. But the student looked uneasy as he picked the card randomly and placed it face down in front of him.

"'So: the queen of clubs?' he said with a defiant smirk.

"'Queen of clubs,' I answered coolly.

"And then he turned over the card and I almost fell off

my chair. It *was* the queen of clubs. I was utterly astonished and didn't speak. The student smiled ruefully and good-naturedly slapped the table, congratulating me on my cabaret trick.

"I have to admit to you, I was as shaken. It really felt like something from M. R. James. I laughed it off, of course, and took the credit as Mandrake the Magician. But it was an interesting moment, a resonant moment. I remember lying awake that night and thinking about all I'd read of the centuries of oral legends about psychokinesis and how we explain it all away now as cognitive bias and illusion."

BASIL FAWLTY

The professor shifted in his chair, amused but not amazed. "It's a nice story, John, but it stinks of trickery and alcohol. I don't think many people would believe you, or the implication of hidden significance. You're confessing to illusion, or self-delusion – but I hear the contradictory note in your voice."

I smiled and asked him about his reading beyond the recognized textbooks of medical study. He had read *Supernature* by Lyall Watson, which argues for the unseen interdependent complexities of the natural world, but, he stressed, he didn't believe a word of that either. I shied away from asking about his knowledge of Darwin, who challenged centuries-old creationism; or Franz Boas, the founder of American anthropology, who tackled scientific racism; or the initiator of quantum physics Max Planck, who modified fundamental aspects of Einstein's immutable laws of physics; or the pioneers of thought experiments like Aldous Huxley, Terence McKenna and Harvard's John E. Mack, whose explorations of the chemistry of the human brain have brought about the reassessments of mind–

body relationship that are being embraced by futurists like Ray Kurzweil, currently at the cutting edge of designing transhuman robotics. "Don't judge too hastily," I told my friend. "I have another story. And this one, you'll be pleased to hear, has no alcohol involved."

"Give it a shot," he said.

My mind rolled back over the years to my personal conversion to the notion of the essential, constant open mind. As a child I was always inquisitive as well as adventurous. Convention only bothered me in one regard: I could never accept the static. The first classroom lesson I learned was the basic truth that history is the lie agreed upon. Contextually much is missed because, as the saying goes, it is the victor who writes the story. Accordingly, logical deduction tells you much is sideswiped and gets lost. When we forensically review cultural history we see the dangers of the poor recording and the omissions. It seems unthinkable that Shakespeare's great works are only 400 years old, yet the records are so bad that we cannot say with certainty that the jobbing actor-playwright called William Shakespeare wrote those immortal plays: it might well have been Lord Oxford, or Christopher Fry, or Ben Jonson; there is circumstantial evidence to support the notion of all of them as alternative authors. There are others in the shadows, like Emmanuel Swedenborg, the modest Swedish scientist who turned away from engineering projects at Uppsala University to devote himself to mystical revelation writing. It is little known that this great visionary was the first scientist to propose the biological and medical importance of the neuron, the hierarchical order of the nervous system, the route of cerebrospinal fluid and the association of the frontal brain regions with the intellect. He was also the first to propose the principles of the formation and development of our solar system, more than 100 years before his theories were verified. With such startling and visionary ingenuity, how has modern culture so comprehensively sidelined Swedenborg? Is it simply because, like Lyall Watson and Huxley, he stepped beyond convention to add spiritual exploration to his portfolio of studies?

My interest in the views of the outsider, from Dostoyevsky to Huxley, turned me to investigating psychosomatic aspects of illness in the 1970s and 1980s. The power of hypnosis and hypnotic suggestion is on our TV screens constantly now, in the person of performers like David Blaine, Paul McKenna and Derren Brown. But my interest was in its medical therapeutic benefits, and so in the 1980s I joined the Irish Society for Clinical and Experimental Hypnosis with the objective of keeping up with developments.

Times and the zeitgeist have changed, but 30 years ago the society was very active and regularly convened to discuss progress of understanding in the various methods being tested worldwide. I was pleased to attend one such meeting in West Cork, where a distinguished guest speaker from the UK was scheduled to lecture on the benefits of Eastern-tradition meditation practices in medicine. An incident at this meeting provided the next story for my sceptical young professor friend. I set the scene by reminding him that hypnosis, though still regarded as entertainment rather than authentic medicine, is paradoxically central to modern psychotherapy practices in several countries.

"Conceded," my friend agreed.

I went on: "Well, our convention was over an autumn weekend, ending late on Sunday afternoon. I had a four-and-a-half-hour drive back to Dublin and was due in work at my surgery as usual on Monday morning. It was all a bit of a rush, and by seven o'clock I was on the back roads but still a long way from connecting with the main highway from Cork to Dublin. Usually on long journeys, like many people, I go on autopilot and generally don't even think about stopping until I reach my final destination. This evening, however, as I was rounding a bend of a country road shortly after seven, I saw a large sign advertising a four-star country house hotel that served dinner. Realizing I hadn't eaten since lunchtime I impulsively turned sharply to the right and was halfway up the long, curving avenue before I knew what I was doing.

"I found it a little odd that there were only two cars in the parking lot at the front of the hotel, but all of the lights in the building were on. When I entered I found nobody at the reception desk and nobody in the lobby. I rang the service bell repeatedly but nobody came. Seeing a sign indicating the dining room, I headed off to look for it. It too was empty. There was nobody there, no guests, no staff and no sign of life. It was all a little eerie and uncomfortable. Since I was pressed for time, I decided to leave and resume the homeward journey. As I made my way back through the empty reception area, suddenly a big man looking very much like Basil Fawlty from the television series came rushing down the stairs. He was dressed in an evening suit complete with a red bowtie. 'I'm sorry, so sorry, so sorry,' he mumbled, rubbing his hands together like a pre-op surgeon. 'I just had to lie down for a few minutes as I had a bit of a sore throat and I didn't hear customers in the lobby. I hope you haven't been waiting too long. So very sorry. I'm having staff problems, you see, a lot of staff problems.' I told him I had stopped for dinner but was in a hurry. Amid a gush of fresh apologies he offered to make me a sandwich. He seemed frantic, discombobulated, so I politely declined. I shook his hand, wished him the best and almost bolted out of the place. My hunger had left me completely by this time.

"I drove straight to Dublin and was home in bed by midnight. In the morning I drove the few miles to my consulting rooms, pleased that my weekend had been mentally refreshing and had readied me for a good week's work. At that time I ran a walk-in surgery in the mornings with only occasional secretarial help. So I was alone and putting my desk in order at 8.45 a.m. when the buzzer from the waiting room sounded. I went out to see who was there. If the President of the United States had been there I couldn't have been more surprised. The person in the waiting room was none other than the previous evening's Basil Fawlty, the hotelkeeper from the periphery of West Cork. He was still in his evening attire, complete with red bowtie. As I was in my surgery coat, with stethoscope about my neck, he looked at me without a trace of recognition. I asked him why he was all dressed up and he told me that he was on his way to an interview for the post of hotel manager at a big Dublin hotel. I smiled, and toyed with the lack of recognition. Just for the fun of it I asked if he had much experience of hotel work. He beamed and told me about the beautiful four-star hotel he'd been managing in West Cork for several years. I pushed the recognition issue, asking had that hotel been busy of late. He wasn't fazed and said, 'Oh, quite, quite. But then there are off-season weekends, like now, when you'd see no one. Well, almost no one.' I waited for a flash of awareness, but there was none. I, then, fell in the category of 'almost no one', it seemed. I just patted his shoulder welcomingly, and got on with the medical check-up.

"As it turned out all he was suffering from was a strep

throat and I gave him some medication and he went on his way. I never saw nor heard from that man again."

My young professor seemed dumbfounded. He gaped expectantly. "I'm sorry, John, but what exactly was the point of this story? Am I to deduce that this is an example of some weird synchronicity implying you are so 'sensitive' that you were drawn to an anonymous hotel in West Cork, picking up distress signals from an ailing manager lying on his bed?"

I laughed. "You tell me. There are 250 kilometres between Dublin and Cork. There are four million people in Ireland. Rural West Cork is relatively sparsely populated. Suburban Dublin, where I have my surgery, is not a densely populated area. You work out that needle-in-a-haystack likelihood. I've been trying to figure it out for years."

"Coincidence?"

"Probably," I said. "Just an incident of extraordinary random happenstance, like the double play on the queen of clubs. Or, if you look at it another way, maybe it was some sort of odd, instinctive communication that made me impulsively drive into this remote hotel just as its manager was deciding to visit a doctor 250 kilometres away 12 hours later."

I saw him raise his eyebrows and squirm in his chair.

I forged on: "Of course, the other explanation is that I simply made up the whole story." I hefted my wine glass. "That it's alcohol talking," I winked.

AN AMERICAN FRIEND COMES CALLING

My young professor huffed and rose to his feet. "I've had enough," he said, but of course he was more amused than annoyed. This was a kind of game for both of us, and I could see there was hesitancy in his every gesture and I knew he was intrigued by the kind of temperament that underlay the passion I was putting into my cancer trials. Like everyone else, I guessed, he had read the exaggerated spooky stories of the sensationalist media and smiled at them with the rest of us. But my anecdotes were touching a different nerve. Our families knew and trusted each other by long association, and he sensed the coherence in the pattern I was indicating.

"No time for just one or two more?" I proposed lightly. When he shuffled his feet I said, "It could be that when I string a few of these incidents together you'll see things differently. Perhaps they'll trigger something that cracks the hard shell of scepticism that insulates specialists like yourself." I was taunting, of course. But I saw I had him. He looked around the room at the scattering of packed tables, friendly folk exchanging banalities about the state of the weather and supermarket prices. Intrigue seemed the better option. He sat back down, sighing resignation but more attentive than before.

"Okay, this is a really short one," I promised. "It's about the time I worked in Mobile, Alabama, almost 50 years ago. I haven't been back there since but when I was there I made many good friends. One of these friends was an orthopaedic surgeon whose house I looked after for some weeks when he was away on vacation. He came to Dublin to visit some 30 years after we'd last met. While we'd departed on the best of terms, there had been no communication in the intervening years. I'd lost his address with the passage of time, and he'd lost mine. As far as he was concerned I might have settled anywhere in the world. Indeed, I might well be dead and buried.

"When he and his wife arrived in Dublin, however, he decided to track me down, since I was an Irishman. He was an optimist and a doer, the kind of positive-thinking American that Norman Vincent Peale coached in his self-help bestsellers. For him, nothing in life was impossible: if you're not in, you can't win was his philosophy. So, settled in his Dublin city hotel, he picked up the telephone directory in his room and looked under 'K' for Kelly.

"To his dismay he found eight small print, three-columned pages full of Kellys, lots and lots of John Kellys and J. Kellys. Had he looked in the business section of the directory he would have found me listed under medical practitioners, of which there were fewer J. Kellys. But he didn't. Others might have abandoned the task, with time short and precious on any vacation. But, with the 'give it a go!' attitude that was typical of him, he simply grabbed the phone and dialled a random John Kelly.

"Now you're probably expecting me to say that the number he called was mine but it's stranger than that. The fact is, at the very moment he was making his phone call I was not at my home but was visiting with my mother. I was seated by her bed, when the telephone rang in the hallway below. She asked me to answer it and tell the person that she would call back. I went down the stairs to do as bidden and almost dropped the receiver when I heard that familiar deep Southern drawl at the other end of the line asking to speak to John Kelly. I recognized that voice immediately and stood frozen on the spot as he, equally amazed, rambled on about the extraordinary coincidence of instant easy contact after 30 silent years. That evening my wife and I had dinner with him and his wife at their city hotel, nattering into the small hours as though resuming an intimate chat from Mobile decades before. The following morning, his vacation over, he and his wife left for the US."

"It sounds like *Tales of the Unexpected*, John. And it's outrageous," the young professor said.

I reflected that he was right. But that incident didn't recall Roald Dahl for me, but rather J. B. Priestley's stories of the mysteries of time. There was no more practical-minded author in Britain in the twentieth century than the North Country Priestley. He was a socialist reformer and the existence of the welfare state owes much to him. He's remembered for his play *An Inspector Calls*, which is a critique of the divisions of social class, but he also wrote about the multi-dimensional probabilities of existence. My young professor friend was reminding me of Priestley's 1940s collection called *The Other Place*, the main story of which is about a man's encounter with a fellow traveller who is fixated on finding a place he knows with certainty exists, even though he believes he's dreamed it. H. G. Wells, that other great social leveller, wrote a similar allegorical story called "The Door in the Wall", about the *other* reality that our instincts tell us is just beyond our comprehension.

"I understand stubborn belief because I am stubborn by nature myself," I told my friend. "But one has always got to check oneself, lest stubbornness becomes self-limiting prejudice. Maybe you are right: maybe these are just good yarns about coincidence. But what if there's more to encounters such as these? What if all those intellectuals, from W. B. Yeats to Colin Wilson, who see patterns in symbols and coincidences are right? I believe we're conditioned to dismiss everything we don't understand and I think we do this at our own peril. Maybe we are prompted all the time by nature. Perhaps my friend from Alabama had a particularly well-developed message-sending mind and perhaps mine was receptive in the best way? Perhaps the synchronicity was a message reminding me of the value of action, no matter how the long-shot odds are stacked against a positive outcome. Who knows, perhaps all those moments were nudging me towards a role of obligation in reading, distilling and promoting the message of Colin Campbell's astonishing findings. It was Goethe who said we open the doors to immense possibilities as soon as we make a decision to act."

THE HOLE IN THE HEART

Incredulity had been replaced by unease and my young friend was on his feet. "Okay, that's it, I'm off! You make a good case, John, but I only believe in empirical facts, in what I can see with my own eyes."

"Like thought?" I said. "Who can *see* thought?"

He fuddled. "You *are* stubborn. But I'm not going to change my mind about your theory on cancer. I guess the word 'alternative' is a blind spot with me."

It was, and its implications kept me seated and focused on his troublesome complacency. Simply, I felt a missionary commitment to stirring up the professional cancer community. The results I was already observing in my own surgery created a moral imperative: I must climb and conquer the walls of rejection; I owed it to my patients and to the countless millions who have faced, or will face, this hideous disease.

I gripped my young friend's arm in the friendliest way. "One last story," I said. "This one features a colleague of yours and you can verify it with him."

"This will convert me to hidden knowledge?" he said sarcastically.

I shook my head. "Regretfully, this one has no happy ending."

He watched me with careful intensity.

"This begins in an Indian restaurant many years back. My wife and I had developed the routine of eating in this particular restaurant every Wednesday evening, and consequently we were known to all the waiters. One waiter in particular had more or less adopted us and ensured that we always got our favourite table. Over the years it had slipped out that I was a doctor so there was often a little chat about his own personal health matters and those of his friends. On this particular evening he had a long, sad face as he told us that his younger brother who lived in Bangladesh had had a baby son but that the child had a hole in his heart. He was close to tears and explained that the baby was almost certain to die as it was impossible to have the necessary heart surgery done in his homeland and the family was too poor to have the surgery done in the UK or Ireland. He queried me as to whether I could arrange to have the operation done under Ireland's free public health system on account of the fact that he, the baby's uncle, had lived in Ireland for seven years. I told him there was little hope but I would inquire. I promised that I would make inquiries and let him know.

"I was depressed for him, and deeply saddened. Experience told me there was nothing I could do and I made a mental note to myself to avoid restaurants where I was known as a medical practitioner, so as to spare myself and others the quandary of hopeless conversations. I did keep my promise to him, however, and made what I'd expected to be a rather embarrassing telephone call to a cardiologist at a Dublin children's hospital. It didn't turn out so bad. Much to my surprise the cardiologist told me that there was a little known clause in the constitution of the hospital that allowed free medical care to be offered to one serious case each year from the Third World. He said that a hole-in-the-heart case from Bangladesh would fit the bill and all I had to do was forward all the medical details for evaluation and a final decision.

"This came as a total surprise to me. Synchronicity had again raised its head. Goethe was right. Action *is* the best policy. I phoned the waiter and told him the good news, which he must relay to his brother. The waiter was beside himself with happiness, even more so when I told him that one or perhaps both parents would be funded to accompany the child. I emphasized the need for the medical files to be forwarded to the children's hospital immediately and I gave him my office telephone number so that he could contact me should there be further queries.

"Giving him my phone number was a rash gesture because within days I was fielding rapid-fire calls from the waiter. Each evening at precisely seven o'clock the telephone would ring and the waiter would make the same inquiries about when the operation would take place, whether both the mother and father would be funded to travel, where the parents might be accommodated, and so on. My responses were always the same: all necessary requirements would be met as soon as the hospital received the medical files. He assured me the files were on the way.

"Weeks passed and the medical notes from Bangladesh never arrived. I was becoming anxious and telephoned the cardiologist to apologize for the delay. The process was under control, I assured him. But it wasn't, and I was becoming increasingly agitated by the repetitive, aimless seven o'clock phone calls, which on many occasions interrupted other patients' consultations in my surgery. Finally, in the middle of a consultation, yet another call came and I stood my ground. I explained firmly to the waiter that I was tied up, that the files were still sought and the best I could do was call him to discuss the following day.

"As I hung up from him I was uneasy. Normally I would never speak to one patient about another's problems but on this particular evening the interrupted patient sitting in front of me happened to be from Washington DC and was just passing through, spending two days in Dublin in transit to somewhere else and looking for a flu remedy. I therefore felt I could relax the rules and explain my exasperation. I told him about the hole-in-the-heart baby in Bangladesh and my dilemma about the files. I was surprised when he suddenly asked me where in Bangladesh the baby lived. I produced the waiter's card with the address written on it and he smiled. 'How strange,' he said. 'I'm going there.' Calmly he proceeded to tell me that he worked for the World Bank and was flying to Bangladesh the very next morning. He also told me that the address written on the card was situated within walking distance of the hotel he stayed at in Bangladesh. If I had never believed in synchronicity I believed in it now. I felt my jaw drop but I recovered quickly enough to if ask if I could impose and request that he visit the child's house to obtain the medical records. He said he would do what he could and we shook hands – and he was gone."

My young professor friend was silent. Long odds, indeed, I guessed he was thinking.

"The medical notes on the baby arrived in my office ten days later and contained some vital information. Not alone did the baby have a hole in the heart, he also suffered from Down syndrome. That fact, I knew, was likely to change everything. I sent the records to the children's hospital and telephoned the cardiologist a few days later. He had already spoken to his colleagues and it had been agreed that surgery on a baby with Down syndrome was not something the hospital was equipped to undertake. With sad regret, the request for intervention would be turned down."

My professor wasn't smiling. "Hard luck stories are much less impressive," he said.

"I chose to end with that for a purpose," I replied. "What I've been recounting amounts to my personal challenge to you, as a friend, to rethink convention. These incidents indicate aspects to our lives that are strange and I think should arouse curiosity in any intelligent person. It isn't about propagating New Age ways of viewing the world. It's about widening our horizons. We could sit here all night recalling crossroads moments in science, in religion, in history where the worldview shifted overnight. We could talk about seemingly overnight breakthroughs, like the discovery of antibiotics, or the polio cure, or the smallpox vaccine. But with reflection we can see that all of these events have a lead-up. Breakthroughs occur, progress comes, because dedicated, coordinated rethinking of a problem is engaged.

"My gripe is that there is insufficient courage or commitment in *coordinated* rethinking of cancer treatment. An extraordinary study, conducted with meticulous care over many years in Oxford University, in Cornell and beyond, has shown a direct link between cancer growth and the consumption of animal protein in foods like meat and dairy products. I'm no fool. I understand the implications are colossal – in terms of new treatment approaches to one of *the* major illnesses, in terms of the food industry, in terms of the pharmaceutical industry, in terms of medical institutional regimes. But the facts *must* be faced and the coordinated follow-up studies and readjustments in care *must* be made. Because, finally, it isn't a medical, or an economic, or a political issue. It is a humanitarian cause."

My friend was now frowning reflectively.

"I told that last story because I wanted us to part with the thought on both our minds of the collateral that's truly involved here. Human beings are robust and complex creatures. As doctors, we are privileged in our vocation because we have duty of care. We are like pilots weighed with the technical and moral responsibility of conveying our human cargo as comfortably as possible to the safe destination. In such a role, complacency is not just irresponsible. It's just plain wrong."

I said goodbye to my young friend shortly after, and we shook hands with affectionate warmth. He was still frowning a little, but I chose to see a chink of change. Maybe, just maybe, the rigours of his training that transformed healthy scepticism into party-line service had been shaken a little. Maybe, just maybe, the baton had been passed. Maybe one new key voice carrying the message would breach the bastions of inaction.

Maybe the conquest of cancer was one step closer.

9

A New Way of Thinking: The Problem of the Pancreas

"Nothing is stronger than an idea whose time has come."
– VICTOR HUGO

It has been my fervent hope in this book to tell a personal story that accurately relates the importance of new findings but does not over-simplify the challenge of cancer. Underestimating the complexity of the disease would be as wrong as overestimating the ease of a universal cure. When my patients query the value of medication in a general sense I always remind them of the time-tested benefits of sound pharmacology. I'm respectful of the decades – indeed centuries – of careful laboratory research that have brought about the powerful treatments we have for so many illnesses today, and I know a good thing when I see it. But pharmacology, like living itself, requires constant re-evaluation and modification, and a by-product of the study that forms the basis of this book has prompted new thoughts about the medical treatment of that most virulent of diseases, cancer of the pancreas.

Let us backtrack. All the case histories that have been presented highlight the close association that exists between the consumption of animal protein and the manner in which the patient's cancer grows. We have been able to show that it is possible to arrest the growth of cancer and that, provided the patient remains compliant with the diet and no serious damage has been inflicted to a vital organ before the diet commenced, the restoration of good health is possible. There can be no exceptions to good scientific theory – or can there be? The question many will ask is, "What about pancreatic cancer?" It's the one that makes most headlines because of its virulent, seemingly unstoppable nature. Everyone has read the media stories – the tragedies of high-profile people like Luciano Pavarotti and the actor Patrick Swayze and so many others who seemingly were cut down in their prime in just months. It is true that cancer of the pancreas has some miserable statistics associated with it. It is the fourth most common cause of cancer-related deaths in the United States and unless it is diagnosed early its survival rate is practically zero. The great problem with this cancer is that very few symptoms are associated with it in the early stages and in most incidences, by the time it is diagnosed, local and metastatic spread has already taken place. It is then too late for surgery which, up till now, has proven the only feasible way to cure a patient.

A reader may well ask have I cherry-picked my patients to make my case in this book? Surely I have come across cases of cancer of the pancreas over the years? What has happened to them? I think I can demonstrate how pancreatic cancer in fact adds to the proof that Colin Campbell's theory is correct. It is the exception that proves the rule.

Over the years of my clinical trials I have been waiting for pancreatic cases to test the animal-protein theory in this regard. As it is not a very common cancer, only four cases came my way during the last decade. I remember all of them in considerable detail as they were all difficult cases that presented very differently from what I had been used to. The story of cancer of the pancreas is very much a story within a story, for although, as we shall discover, it too has a close association with animal protein, I soon learned it was not possible to stop these cancers from growing by simply limiting the amount of animal protein in the diet.

I encountered my first case of pancreatic cancer 18 months into my clinical trial. I was checking a lady for possible gallstones when an ultrasound detected a malignant lesion in the pancreas. This came as a major shock to my patient, of course, but since the scan showed the cancer had not spread beyond its original site, the surgeon I referred her to was of the opinion that the cancer might be curable. I added my contribution to that heartening news by telling her enthusiastically about *The China Study* and the value of assuming an animal-protein-free diet.

Within a few days the surgery had been performed and the surgeon was confident that the cancer had been entirely removed. Her recovery was uneventful, and when she was discharged from hospital a short while later she telephoned to thank me for sending her to that particular surgeon and to say she was enjoying the new diet. At that time my only "gripe" was the speed of resolution; everything had gone so remarkably well that I felt the case hardly rated as a particularly good test of Colin Campbell's theory. Still, I chalked it up as a great victory and was very happy for my recovering patient.

Two months later, however, there was some bad news. A letter from the surgeon informed me that a new focus of the cancer had been discovered within the pancreas and that the patient was now undergoing chemotherapy. Three months later, she was dead.

It was a shock. My belief was that, whether the cancer that killed her was the recurrence of the original or a completely new tumour, it should not have happened while the patient was on the diet. On the face of it at that time, I confess, this appeared to be a setback for Campbell's theory. As the patient was deceased I couldn't question her about how compliant she'd been with diet. Such was my own belief in its efficacy and such was the long string of successes I'd had up till then that I felt fairly sure this may have been the root problem. I had, after all, seen the terrible results when over-confident recovering patients abandoned the diet. I was also aware that, since my patient was under the care of hospital doctors after her follow-up surgery, it was unlikely she'd been carefully guided on the dietary issues. The awful truth for the patient was that she got no second chance.

A couple of years passed before I had my next case of pancreatic cancer. A man aged 65 had been attending a gastroenterologist with abdominal pain and a cancer had been discovered at the head of the pancreas. As with my previous case, this cancer did not appear to have spread beyond the primary site, and the surgeon was once again quite optimistic. This time I took extra time and care with the patient before he was admitted to hospital to explain to him the importance of the diet. To encourage compliance, I told him about the previous case and my suspicions of a lapse in adherence. He listened attentively and said he was determined to take the advice and make sure the same fate didn't befall him. What transpired, however, was totally unexpected. On the night before the surgery was due to take place, to the consternation of everyone, a massive haemorrhage occurred at the cancer site and, in spite of all efforts by the best medical staff, the patient died.

If nothing else, this incident was a dramatic demonstration of the aggressiveness of pancreatic cancer; there was clearly no one to blame for what had happened. But in a way I blamed myself. I regretted that the patient had not been on the diet a little longer, theorising that this may have lessened the aggression of the cancer and stopped the haemorrhage. I had some sleepless nights. All I could think of was that I had only come across two cases of pancreatic cancer and I had lost both my patients. If only I'd gotten the message of the association between animal protein and cancer across to the medical profession more quickly and conclusively, I felt, these tragedies might not have unfolded.

I took comfort from the progress of the other patients in my trial, but the pancreas issue was never far from my thoughts. I had to wait three years before another pancreatic case presented itself. In fact, two showed up in quick succession. There were striking similarities between the cases. Both were males between 60 and 70 years old, both had extensive metastatic spread by the time of diagnosis, and tragically both patients were dead within a few months, the agony of their final weeks barely controlled by high doses of pain-killing drugs. The last patient to die was my own brother, who was eight years my junior.

Observing a family member's death in such pain from this most vigorous cancer was a horrific experience. The anguish seemed worse since he'd known all about Colin Campbell's work and told me he'd been following the animal-protein-free diet. I do not know how disciplined he was with the diet but, knowing him so well, I suspect he was at least reasonably so. I was heartbroken, but his death focused my mind as never before. I had studied every aspect accessible to me about cancer and I felt sure there was a fundamental difference between cancer of the pancreas and other cancers. I reread everything I could about the disease, and scoured the Internet daily to make sure I wasn't missing anything. I went to sleep thinking about pancreatic cancer, and woke every morning still thinking of it. Then came my eureka moment, a flash of clarity.

As with so many eureka moments a simple answer proposed itself. My deduction, based on all the published and known scientific facts, was that in cancer of the pancreas it wasn't the dietary animal protein that was most relevant, but rather the structure and function of the pancreas itself. In the unique case of the pancreas, its own cells – and any cancers therein – have the ability *to produce their own animal protein already fully metabolized* and ready for use. What I had overlooked was the fact that more than 90 per cent of pancreatic cancers take place in the glandular cells of the pancreas and that the normal function of these cells is to produce the enzymes that metabolize the foods we eat. The enzyme involved in metabolizing protein – the culprit we are interested in – is called trypsin.

Trypsin is produced by the glandular cells of the pancreas and is stored there in an inactive form (trypsinogen) until there is need for it. When we eat protein it is fed into the upper part of the small intestine, where it becomes active and thus capable of metabolizing the consumed proteins so they can be absorbed into the bloodstream and utilized by the body. Trypsin is a very powerful enzyme and the reason it is normally stored in the inactive state is that it might otherwise begin to metabolize and corrupt the pancreatic cells themselves. In fact, this sometimes does occur, in a nonmalignant condition called pancreatitis where self-digestion results in inflammation and destruction of pancreatic cells. This is a condition often associated with chronic alcohol abuse.

Trypsin does not cause cancer. But what my eureka moment suggested was that should a number of pancreatic cells begin malignant change – for whatever reason – the trypsin produced by these cells could trigger auto-digestion of the protein structure within the cell, thereby providing an endless supply of best-quality animal protein that would nourish rapidly replicating, rapidly metastasizing cancer cells indefinitely. Small wonder, then, that it is virtually impossible to cure pancreatic cancer once the surgical option of removing a localized tumour is no longer feasible.

It must be mentioned that cancer of the stomach provides a similar cellular scenario to that of the pancreas. In this instance, the glandular cells of the stomach produce an enzyme called pepsin, which is also involved in metabolizing protein. In the event that some of these cells become cancerous, the pepsin might prompt a similar state of auto-digestion that feeds widespread cancer growth. So similar are the cancers of the glandular cells of the stomach and the pancreas that, in the case of my brother, his doctors were never quite certain which organ contained the primary lesion. Finally, it hardly mattered. Given the treatments applied, which today represent the very best of clinical care, the result would have been the same.

I believe we have approached a critical border here. If my deduction is right, we are broaching a broad range of new possibilities that might be of considerable importance in new treatments for cancers of the pancreas and stomach, and perhaps all cancers. The role played by trypsin and pepsin in feeding the worst cancers has been too long overlooked because nobody has pressed the argument that a devastating association between animal protein and cancer growth exists. Now that it is becoming clear that such a link does exist, these enzymes must come under renewed scrutiny. It is my view that oncology experts should lead the field in reviewing the role of the anti-trypsin chemicals that we know exist naturally in the body, but I believe it is quite likely that the pharmaceutical industry will step up the pace, and hugely effective medications will result. The process of producing these drugs might turn out to be easier than anyone expects because, as I say, both anti-trypsin and anti-pepsin occur naturally.

In the end it may well be that all that's required to finally defeat pancreatic and stomach cancer, indeed all cancers, is an anti-trypsin and anti-pepsin medication available at the bedside.

Epilogue

No wars are won in a single action. It takes vision, courage and coordinated planning to overcome the odds and resolve the conflict. To maintain the analogy, I see Colin Campbell's work as visionary and, like the courier carrying notes in the battlefield, I see myself, as I said at the start of this book, as a messenger. So while this book lacks commercial calculation it openly admits to a hard publishing strategy: Cancer is a pervasive, stubborn and terrible disease, but we, all of us, have the proven knowledge of a new method to tackle it and the onus is on everyone to participate in a fundamental change of mindset.

It may be perceived that I skipped somewhat lightly over the economic fallout of a major rethinking of what constitutes what we now know to be the safe human diet. Inevitably, cultural changes will affect the food industry, perhaps even more dramatically than the business of pharmaceutical production. Professor Campbell is not shy about stating that a great deal of opposition to his ideas of an altered diet has come from Big Business. He accuses the food industry of having frequently employed its own "experts" to supply what he considers dubious statistics, and even of stooping to infiltrating distinguished scientific committees set up by government agencies with the brief of improving the American diet in order to reduce health care costs. Industrial espionage and skilled lobbying are only part of the story, says Campbell. "Company men" insinuated onto research committees ensured that the security of economic interests was prioritized by blocking critical research funding for scientists known to be engaged in projects deemed contrary to the interests of the food industry.

You may ask here what further critical research needs to be done. It's an important question. Professor Campbell has established beyond doubt the fact that animal protein exacerbates cancerous cell growth. Animal protein is an essential food for cancers. As I mentioned earlier, vital work has been done by the Harvard School of Public Health and by EPIC, under the auspices of the World Health Organization. But more specific, *unified*, targeted laboratory studies are needed to investigate the subdivisions of our definition of animal protein. Processed meat, it is clear from almost all studies, is a no-go. But is chicken/fowl protein precisely as troublesome as red meat? All indications drawn from *The China Study* suggest fish protein has no effect at all on cancer cell growth, but this requires further extensive laboratory research. In my view the leaders of Big Business would gain immense advantage, not only politically but also morally, by taking the lead in advancing such research. In the short term, investment in shaking up our food biases might seem detrimental for them. In the long term they would benefit. As the old saying goes, change happens whether one likes it or not; so, perhaps far better to be driving change than burying one's head in the ground like the proverbial ignorant ostrich.

There is a recent precedent to suggest that the true impact of redoubled animal-protein studies might be much less disruptive for the food industry than the doomsayer economists think. In the middle of the twentieth century a seemingly insurmountable threat faced dairy farming when it was discovered that the cholesterol contained in milk, cheese, cream and butter was, beyond question, a major factor in coronary heart disease. Most people who lived through that era will remember how events unfolded. The food industry at first attempted to ignore the whole matter, but the relentlessness of rolling news reports and the avalanche of corroborative statistics finally presented an unavoidable challenge. Business was *forced* to respond. Within a very short time supermarket shelves worldwide were packed with ranges of new foods from which all or most of the cholesterol had been removed. Then the business domino effect kicked in. The pharmaceutical industry followed suit by introducing new, low-cost medications capable of limiting the amount of cholesterol in the blood stream. Cynicism quickly turned to celebratory self-congratulation. Through the aggressive action of food and drug suppliers the rates of coronary heart disease in numerous countries were dramatically reduced. In the end everybody was a winner. The food producers made happy profits from new, alternative, safer products; the drug manufacturers widened their brand ranges; and international health standards and disease survival rates improved.

The world *is* changing. Instant media and the power of the Internet means facts travel faster. Established ideas in all disciplines face scrutiny every day – and this is socially beneficial as new ideas emerge faster, are tested faster, and displace the jaded status quo. When we look back at the recent decades we see how fast and effective change can be.

Veganism and a holistic approach to living were virtually underground movements in the 1960s. They are now considered mainstream practices, veering month by month from the fetish stain of "fringe fads" to noble pursuits assured to lengthen and improve quality of life. This confluence of factors – awareness of business benefit, transparency and urgency of investigative news, the embracing of a holistic approach to health – paves the ground perfectly for a concentrated worldwide follow-up to the lessons of *The China Study*.

In the end, though, I am a realist. I don't believe the ultimate change will come from Big Business or the go-getters leading investigative reports on the nightly news. The revolution is likely to come from those who have the most to gain by changing direction – from those who adopt an animal-protein-free diet and experience the immediate benefit. There is no magic in the "cure" of course. In cases where cancer has already caused irreparable damage to vital organs, different remedial support needs will still apply. But to others suffering onset cancer, adherence to the animal-protein-free diet will be a blessing: they can look forward to feeling better within weeks. These are the people I have the most faith in as the ultimate change-makers. Bit by bit, I believe, their revolutionary experiences will emerge into the daylight of common knowledge, and the blight of cancer will be seen differently.

Ultimately we are all in Professor Colin Campbell's debt. My informal study – the work outlined in this modest autobiographical book – leaves me in no doubt of the groundbreaking significance of what Campbell has achieved. He will be seen in future years as the father of a revolution comparable, perhaps, to Jonas Salk, whose radical polio treatment policy was once viewed (albeit briefly) with suspicion. It will be seen that Campbell's research let a wondrous genie out of the bottle. My role and the role of everybody who goes on the diet is to spread the word. The sharing of stories of recovery by word of mouth will result in saving the lives of many more people, and each person who spreads the word should remember they are driving a revolution.

A final word – or rather, a pleading restatement: this book serves not only as a hopeful address to those affected by cancer. It is a sincere plea to the medical profession to unify in pushing all resources, institutionally, financially and in manpower, to speed the last phase of research necessary to prove beyond any measure of doubt the direct link between an animal-protein diet and human cancer. To my medical colleagues whom I have caused offence, please know none was intended. I am duty bound to share the truth of what I have in my fieldwork been privileged to see, record and learn from. This information is far too important to bury out of a sense of complicit collegiality.

I trust that the patients who take advantage of the animal-protein-free diet will stay true to their aim, and that their many stories of recovery will inspire the relevant research and institutional change that is now overdue. The tools to defeat one of humanity's greatest scourges are in your hands.

Acknowledgement

I would like to acknowledge the contribution made by Gillian Demurtas in helping me put this book together. Over the past four years her constant encouragement and considerable writing skills enabled me to persevere with my endeavour and in a very real sense were responsible for this book finally seeing the light of day. I thank her for that.

Appendix 1

RECOMMENDED BOOKS

This book clearly isn't a dietary advice book. But for those suffering from cancer, or with a family history of predisposition to the disease, I cannot recommend highly enough the following books.

Beat Cancer: How to Control Your Health and Your Life by Jane Plant CBE and Mustafa Djamgoz (Vermilion, London, 2014)

The Plant Progamme: Recipes for Fighting Breast and Prostate Cancer by Jane Plant CBE and Gillian Tidey (Virgin Books/ Random House, London, 2004)

Anticancer: A New Way of Life by David Servan-Schreiber (Michael Joseph, London, 2011)

The China Study Cookbook by Leanne Campbell, PhD (BenBella Books, Dallas, 2013)

Whole: Rethinking the Science of Nutrition by T. Colin Campbell (BenBella Books, Dallas, 2014)

And finally, of course, I must refer one and all to the book that inspired this book, in the hope that you too will find the magic in its pages:

The China Study by T. Colin Campbell (BenBella Books, Dallas, 2006)

Appendix 2

PRESS ASSOCIATION RELEASE

5 March 2014

High-protein Diet Could be as Dangerous as Smoking – Study

A high-protein diet could be as dangerous as smoking 20 cigarettes a day, a new study has found.

Research from the University of Southern California shows that high levels of dietary animal protein in those under 65 were associated with a fourfold increase in their risk of death from cancer compared to those on a low-protein diet.

This is an increased mortality risk associated with a 20-a-day smoking habit.

The study of 6,318 adults over the age of 50, found that protein-lovers were 74 per cent more susceptible to early death from any cause than their low-protein counterparts. They were also several times more likely to die of diabetes.

A "high-protein" diet was defined in the research as deriving at least 20 per cent of daily calories from protein. The researchers recommend a middle-aged person consume around 0.8g of protein per kilogram of body weight, per day.

Even small changes that reduced someone's protein intake from moderate to low levels cut the likelihood of an early death by over a fifth. A "low-protein" diet includes less than 10 per cent of your daily calorie intake from protein.

Animal-based proteins such as red meat, milk, and cheese were most harmful, but there is no evidence to suggest that protein from fish has a negative impact on the body, said study author Dr Valter Longo, Professor of Biogerontology at the USC Davis School of Gerontology.

"High levels of protein can be as bad for you as smoking. People should understand the distinction and be able to make the decision about what they eat," said Dr Longo.

"Some proteins are better for you than others, for example plant-based proteins like beans. Vegans seem to do better in studies than those who eat animal-based proteins. Red meat always comes out top as the worst and that's probably due to its other components."

"But the good news is that there is no evidence that fish is bad for you. So fish plus vegetables is really the best group of proteins," added Dr Longo.

The findings throw doubt over the long-term benefits of popular high-protein diets such as the Atkins diet and the Paleo diet.

Protein levels control the growth hormone IGF-I, which help bodies grow but high levels of which have been linked to cancer.

Levels of IGF-I drop off dramatically after age 65, leading to potential frailty and muscle loss. The study shows that while high-protein intake during middle age is very harmful, it is protective for those over 65 who ate a moderate or high-protein diet.

Dr Longo, who skips lunch, recommends a diet high in complex carbohydrates and low in protein.

"I follow a fish- and vegetable-based diet which is high in complex carbohydrates. This is a diet that has been found in the most long-lived populations of the world," he said.